HYPERTENSION
A Practical Approach

MURRAY EPSTEIN, M.D.
Professor of Medicine, University of Miami
School of Medicine and Veterans Administration
Medical Center, Miami, Florida

JAMES R. OSTER, M.D.
Associate Professor of Medicine, University of
Miami School of Medicine and Veterans Administration
Medical Center, Miami, Florida

W. B. SAUNDERS COMPANY
Philadelphia • London • Toronto • Mexico City • Rio de Janeiro • Sydney • Tokyo

W. B. Saunders Company: West Washington Square
Philadelphia, PA   19105

1 St. Anne's Road
Eastbourne, East Sussex BN21 3UN, England

1 Goldthorne Avenue
Toronto, Ontario M8Z 5T9, Canada

Apartado 26370—Cedro 512
Mexico 4, D.F., Mexico

Rua Coronel Cabrita, 8
Sao Cristovao Caixa Postal 21176
Rio de Janeiro, Brazil

9 Waltham Street
Artarmon, N.S.W. 2064, Australia

Ichibancho, Central Bldg., 22-1 Ichibancho
Chiyoda-Ku, Tokyo 102, Japan

Library of Congress Cataloging in Publication Data

Epstein, Murray.

Hypertension, a practical approach.

1. Hypertension.   I. Oster, James R.   II. Title. [DNLM:
   1. Hypertension. WG 340 E645h]

RC685.H8E65 1984   616.1'32   83–14290

ISBN 0–7216–3397–8

HYPERTENSION–A Practical Approach   ISBN   0-7216-3397-8

Last digit is the print number: 9   8   7   6   5   4   3   2

To our wives
Nina Epstein and Sharon Oster
and
To our children
David and Susanna Epstein and Marc, Harold and Jacqueline Oster

Preface

The historic report of Freis and associates in 1967 demonstrated in compelling fashion that therapeutic intervention in patients with severe hypertension decreased morbidity and mortality. Their findings represented a watershed in the management of this disease. Subsequently, the medical profession throughout the world invested enormous amounts of time, energy, and intellectual endeavor in further defining the vagaries of hypertension, extending our understanding of its pathophysiology, and establishing new and more appropriate therapeutic regimens.

Many books deal with all aspects of hypertension, but several tend to overwhelm or discourage the clinician who does not specialize in nephrology, cardiology, or hypertension—either by their encyclopedic format or their esoteric orientation.

This book has been developed to assist the primary care physician or internist who wishes to deepen his understanding of hypertension and to broaden his skills in managing patients with this disease. In a real sense, this is intended to be a "how-to" book in regard to both the diagnosis and the treatment of hypertension. We have attempted to present a middle course between the encyclopedic monographs on hypertension and the necessarily brief and more general coverage offered by standard textbooks of internal medicine. Sources and material not readily available to the practicing physician have been culled and collated for ready access.

Although this book is intended primarily for physicians, we believe that it will also prove to be useful to medical students and to the paramedical professional engaged either directly or peripherally in the care of the hypertensive patient.

In preparing this text, we imposed on the friendship of expert colleagues, who reviewed and criticized each chapter. Their skill, interest, and willingness to help are greatly appreciated: Drs. Marshall D. Lindheimer, Meyer D. Lifschitz, Solomon Papper, Lawrence M. Fishman, Andrew Taylor, and Ralph H. Aden, and Ellen Green, M.S., R.D.

Our deep gratitude goes to two fine ladies—Mses. Tam M. Eggers and Jacqueline Sheets—who provided excellent secretarial support, and to Lorraine Kilmer and her associates at Saunders, whose skills are beyond praise.

Finally, we would like to express our deep gratitude to our wives for their continued support and encouragement in helping us see this undertaking through from concept to publication.

MURRAY EPSTEIN

JAMES R. OSTER

NOTE ON DOSAGE OF MEDICATIONS

Although every attempt has been made to provide accurate and current dosage schedules and listings of adverse reactions in this book, it is possible that they may change. Therefore, the reader is urged to review the package informational data of the manufacturers of the medications mentioned in this book.

THE AUTHORS

Contents

I

Natural History and Evaluation of Hypertension

1
WHAT IS HYPERTENSION?

Hypertension is one of mankind's most common diseases, affecting 15 to 20 per cent of all adult Americans. Furthermore, cardiovascular disease associated with hypertension constitutes a leading cause of both mortality and morbidity in the United States. In recent years, physicians and scientists have mounted a concerted effort to define the mechanisms responsible for high blood pressure and to design increasingly more effective approaches to therapy. Such efforts have been encouraged by abundant evidence that successful control of hypertension leads to diminished morbidity and mortality from stroke, heart disease, and, perhaps, renal failure. Perhaps the hallmark studies in this context were the early Veterans Administration Cooperative Studies on Antihypertensive Agents, which provided the first well-documented evidence that lowering blood pressure is of significant value in reducing the cardiovascular hazards of untreated hypertension. Clearly, it is imperative for the physician to attempt to identify and treat patients with hypertension in the general population.

Hypertension is accepted as one of the major disease states afflicting the population, but there is still debate regarding the level of blood pressure that is abnormally high. One renowned authority, Sir George Pickering, emphasized that there is no arbitrary dividing line between "normal" and "high" blood pressure. Rather, he argued that the relationship between arterial pressure and morbidity is quantitative: the higher the pressure, the worse the prognosis. In spite of the arbitrariness of dealing with exact figures, the setting of standards is necessary, since decisions regarding diagnostic evaluation and initiation of therapy must be predicated on some rational basis. Realizing that many "official" criteria are set without provision for such variables as the age and the sex of the patients, we would like to propose the following definition for definite hypertension, which is adapted from Kaplan:

Men under 45	130/90 mm Hg
Men over 45	140/95 mm Hg
Women	160/95 mm Hg

Aside from defining hypertension, it is often useful from an operational standpoint to categorize hypertensive patients according to the severity of their elevated blood pressure. We recommend the arbitrary guidelines shown in

TABLE 1–1. SEVERITY OF HYPERTENSION

Severity	Diastolic BP	Systolic BP
Borderline	84–89 mm Hg	128–146 mm Hg
Mild	90–104 mm Hg	147–159 mm Hg
Moderate	105–114 mm Hg	160–180 mm Hg
Severe	Greater than 114 mm Hg	Greater than 180 mm Hg

Table 1–1 for classifying patients as having borderline, mild, moderate, or severe hypertension. Even though the risk to an individual patient does not necessarily correlate with the severity of his blood pressure elevation, such a schema is helpful in deciding whom to treat and how vigorously.

In considering the evaluation of a patient with hypertension, one should remember that the two principal forms differ greatly in prevalence. Hypertension is arbitrarily classified as being either *essential* or *secondary*. The former diagnosis is established by exclusion of identifiable secondary causes. *Essential hypertension*, the pathogenesis of which is still uncertain, accounts for approximately 95 per cent of cases in adult Americans and will be dealt with in Chapter 2. *Secondary hypertension*, implying a discernible and sometimes reversible *cause* for the elevated blood pressure, probably accounts for less than 5 per cent of cases and will be discussed in Chapter 3.

DETERMINING THE BLOOD PRESSURE

The initial step in management of the patient with suspected hypertension is documenting the presence of hypertension. Yet this seemingly simple maneuver is fraught with potential difficulties. Many blood pressure readings are incorrect, primarily because of two major problems: (a) controversy as to what constitutes a proper setting in which to obtain a "true" reading and (b) errors in measurement.

Proper Setting

Even though there is disagreement over whether a casual or an early morning basal pressure should be used, most clinicians agree that a casual blood pressure taken in the office is quite adequate, providing that a few simple precautions are adhered to (Table 1–2).

First, since blood pressure varies throughout the day (and indeed may vary seasonally), no patient should be labeled as hypertensive on the basis of one blood pressure reading. Rather, several determinations should be made over the period of a few days to several weeks, depending on the level of the pressure.

The clinician should be aware of a phenomenon termed "regression to the mean." This is a statistical term referring to the observation that the more often the blood pressure is taken, the more the pressure approaches that person's average reading. To look at it another way, with repetition, one is less likely to obtain the outlying higher or lower blood pressure values.

At any given visit an average of three blood pressure readings taken at least two minutes apart is preferable to the use of only one reading. Not infrequently, the first reading is unduly high, perhaps related to patient anxiety. Initially, it is worthwhile to determine the blood pressure in both the lying and sitting position, since certain conditions such as pheochromocytoma may be

TABLE 1–2. CONSIDERATIONS IN IMPROVING THE VALUE OF CASUAL BLOOD PRESSURE READINGS

1. Several determinations should be made over a period of a few to several weeks depending on the level of hypertension.
2. The patient should rest quietly for at least five minutes before measurement.
3. Factors that perturb the blood pressure should be avoided, including the following:
   a. Anxiety or pain
   b. Recent eating or smoking
   c. Recent exercise
   d. Cold
   e. Talking or performing mental calculations
   f. Bladder distention
   g. Medications
      (1) Sympathomimetic agents such as nasal drops or sprays, mydriatrics, cold remedies, appetite depressants, or methylphenidate
      (2) Adrenal corticosteroids
      (3) Estrogens

associated with marked posture-related differences. Once pharmacologic therapy has been initiated, this procedure is again indicated, especially if the antihypertensive agent has a tendency to produce postural hypotension. On the first visit only, the patient's pressure should be checked in both arms and in one leg to avoid missing the diagnosis of coarctation of the aorta or subclavian artery stenosis.

The patient should rest quietly in a pleasant setting for at least five minutes before the initial blood pressure determination. Several factors that may elevate the blood pressure and confound interpretation of the readings should be avoided. They include anxiety, eating, smoking, pain, talking or calculating during the actual measurement and the recent use of sympathomimetic agents (Table 1–2). The arm muscles should be relaxed and the forearm supported. A suitable cuff is applied firmly and evenly to the exposed upper arm, with care taken to avoid tight sleeves.

Causes of Error

There are several potential procedural and technical mistakes that can result in erroneous blood pressure readings (Table 1–3).

The mercury sphygmomanometer is the standard simple instrument for measuring blood pressure against which all other methods are compared (the very units of blood pressure, of course, are given in mm Hg). It is very uncommon for anything to be amiss with the mercury manometer per se, yet the instrument should be checked periodically to ensure that the mercury reservoir is full, that the glass column is clean, and that the air hole at the top is patent so that the mercury may fall freely. Anercid devices, of course, must be properly calibrated by the manufacturer before use and should be periodically recalibrated against a mercury manometer, depending on the frequency of use and the care given to the instrument. If the needle does not register 0 mm Hg with the cuff uninflated, considerable error may result.

Improperly sized arm cuffs may present a problem. Although some controversy surrounds this issue, the most important potential source of inaccuracy is the use of a cuff with too short a balloon, resulting unpredictably

**TABLE 1–3. CAUSES OF OBSERVER OR MECHANICAL ERROR IN BLOOD
PRESSURE DETERMINATION**

1. Inappropriate equipment
   a. Improper arm cuff (too short and/or too narrow)
   b. Faulty measuring device
      (a) Aneroid needle not registering 0 mm Hg with the cuff uninflated
      (b) Failure to calibrate aneroid periodically against mercury
          manometer
      (c) Too little mercury in sphygmomanometer
      (d) Dirt on glass column
      (e) Blockage of air hole
2. Erroneous determinations
   a. Improper placement of cuff on arm
   b. Failure to appreciate auscultatory gap
   c. Failure to appreciate or specify the difference between phase IV
      versus V of the diastolic blood pressure
   d. Improper inflation or deflation of cuff, i.e. either overly rapid or
      excessive inflation or excessively slow deflation
   e. Arrhythmias with marked pulse irregularities
   f. Observer bias

in artifactually high readings. Figure 1–1 depicts the influence of arm circumference on blood pressure measurements in normal subjects using different size cuffs. As is evident, use of the two cuffs whose length was only 26 cm was associated with falsely elevated readings when the arm circumference was greater than 28 to 31 cm.

We agree with The World Health Organization recommendation that a cuff with a longer balloon be used if the circumference of a patient's arm exceeds 30 cm. It has been suggested that the width of the balloon assumes importance only if the balloon is also too short, in which case a narrow cuff will also tend to produce erroneously high pressures. In *general*, no harm can arise from the use of the longer, wider cuff in virtually every *adult* patient regardless of arm dimension. When a larger cuff is not available, sometimes a regular-sized cuff can be applied to the forearm and the stethoscope placed over the radial artery.

Errors may arise from faulty techniques as well as from faulty equipment. For example, the cuff might not be placed at heart level, or one might fail to appreciate either the auscultatory gap or a large difference between phases four and five of the diastolic blood pressure.

In 1905, Korotkoff reported the auscultatory phenomena below the cuff that Riva-Rocci had described nine years previously. These Korotkoff sounds cover an average range of 45 mm Hg, which is subdivided into five phases of variable duration:

    I. A loud, clear-cut snapping tone (14 mm Hg)
   II. A succession of murmurs (20 mm Hg)
  III. A duller snapping tone (5 mm Hg)
  IV. A muffled tone (6 mm Hg)
   V. A disappearance of all sounds

Despite much investigation, there is still disagreement over whether phase IV or phase V correlates best with the *true* diastolic blood pressure as measured by direct intra-arterial recording. This may mean that with the current state of knowledge neither criterion is more accurate or yields a smaller systematic

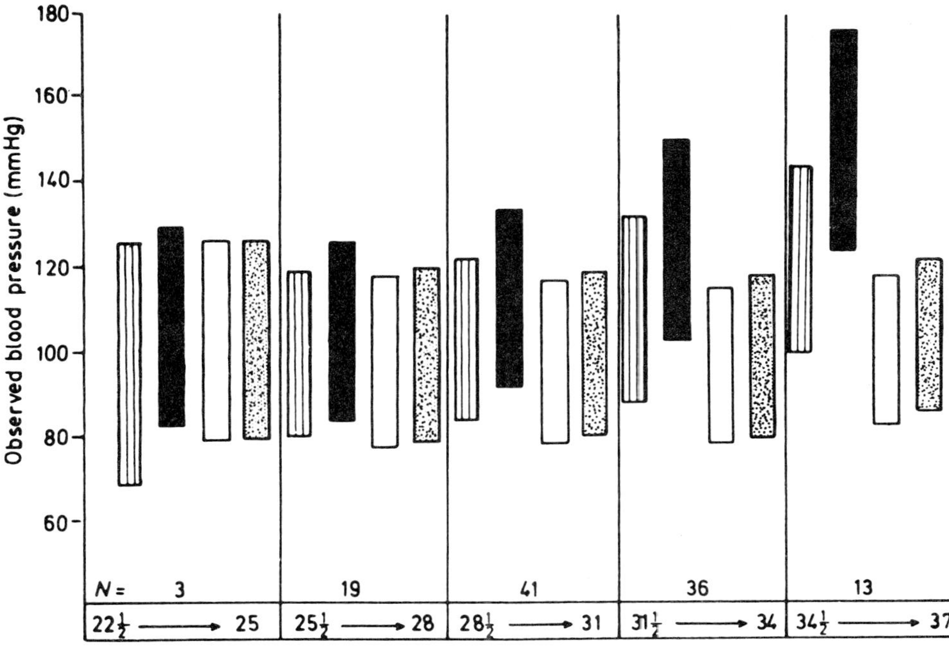

FIGURE 1–1. The influence of arm circumference on blood pressure measurements in normal subjects using different-sized cuffs. As can be seen, when the arm circumference exceeded 28 to 31 cm, the use of the two cuffs whose length was only 26 cm was associated with falsely elevated readings. (Reproduced with permission from King, GE: Clin Sci 32:229, 1967.)

error. An important point, however, is the recent documentation that phase V readings have a smaller random variance and result in the best interobserver agreement. Although these observations certainly commend the use of phase V, the recommendation of the World Health Organization to record the levels of both phases, for example, 140/80–70 mm Hg, especially when the difference between them is greater than 5 mm Hg, makes good sense.

As noted in a study of 275 subjects, there is a difference in the ease of determining phase IV versus phase V in children and adults. In adults, unless a high output state such as aortic insufficiency or severe anemia is present, phase V may be appreciated in virtually every patient, whereas phase IV may be ascertained in only about 55 per cent of patients. In contrast, muffling is more frequent in children (84 per cent), and disappearance is heard in only 73 per cent.

If the blood pressure cuff is inflated excessively, the discomfort produced might elevate the pressure. Rarely, excessively slow deflation might lead to arterial spasm and inaccurately high pressures. If the cuff is deflated too rapidly, the observer tends to underestimate the readings. Arrhythmias with marked pulse irregularities make blood pressure recording difficult. Finally, observer bias can lead to error. Substantial (5 to 10 mm Hg) and consistent variations of blood pressure readings may occur between different observers. These may be related to faulty technique, hearing loss, inaccurate interpretation of Korotkoff sounds, preconceived ideas of important levels, bias from past readings, or concern for other considerations such as the patient's eligibility for life insurance. Obviously, observer preference for certain terminal digits, such as 5 or 0, may also produce inaccuracies.

TABLE 1–4. INDICATIONS FOR DETERMINATION OF BLOOD PRESSURE AT HOME

1. Marked lability of blood pressure
2. Sizable discrepancy between blood pressure readings inside and outside the physician's office
3. Poor control of blood pressure, particularly in association with hypotensive symptoms
4. As an aid for self-medication or dosage adjustment
5. As an aid to compliance in certain patients

A rare cause of potentially serious inaccuracy is based on the fact that blood pressure measurement by the indirect method used clinically (as opposed to direct measurement requiring arterial puncture) requires complete occlusion of the artery by the cuff. Patients with markedly thickened and sometimes calcified arteries (Monckeberg's sclerosis), whose brachial arteries cannot be compressed, may appear to have blood pressures as high as 300/200 mm Hg despite the administration of nitroprusside. This phenomenon has been termed pseudohypertension. We have seen one such patient whose intra-arterial pressure was measured and found to be 60/10 mm Hg. (Also see case study 1.)

HOME BLOOD PRESSURES

The values of and indications for home blood pressure recordings are still somewhat controversial (Table 1–4). Obviously, home blood pressures are not necessary in the vast majority of hypertensive subjects. In fact, when blood pressure control is excellent, there is little reason to get additional readings, and some anxious patients do better when not continuously reminded about their hypertension. On the other hand, home blood pressure recording can prove helpful in patients with marked lability of blood pressure, particularly if it turns out that the pressures are elevated only in the doctor's office (so-called office hypertension). Additional advantages may obtain in patients with very poor blood pressure control as an aid to readjustment of dosing or timing of drug administration. Finally, certain patients become more compliant when asked to take part in their own care by recording their blood pressures in a systematic fashion.

*REFERENCES**

Kaplan, NM: Clinical Hypertension, 3rd ed. The Williams & Wilkins Co., Baltimore, 1982.
Pickering, GW: High Blood Pressure. Churchill, London, 1968.
Pickering, G: Hypertension. Definitions, natural histories and consequences. Am J Med 52:570–583, 1972.
Horan, MC, Kennedy, HL, and Padgett, NE: Do borderline hypertensive patients have labile blood pressure? Ann Intern Med 94:466–468, 1981.
Kannel, WB, Sorlie, P, and Gordon, T: Labile hypertension: A faulty concept? The Framingham Study. Circulation 61:1183–1187, 1980.
Drayer, JIM, Weber, MA, DeYoung, JL, and Wyle, FA: Circadian blood pressure patterns in ambulatory hypertensive patients. Am J Med 73:493–500, 1982.

---

*For simplicity and easy reading, we have made no attempt to be all-inclusive with regard to references and have not cited them directly in the text. Rather a limited number of important and current references are cited at the end of each chapter. These follow the sequence of subject matter within the chapters and in many instances are subdivided by headings.

Taking the Blood Pressure

King, GE: Errors in clinical measurement of blood pressure in obesity. Clin Sci 32:223–237, 1967.

King, GE: Taking the blood pressure. JAMA 209:1902–1904, 1969.

Webb, CH: The measurement of blood pressure and its interpretation. Primary Care 7:637–651, 1980.

Kirkendall, WM, Burton, AC, Epstein, FH, and Freis, ED: Recommendations for human blood pressure determination by sphygmomanometers. Circulation 36:980–988, 1967.

Short, D: The diastolic dilemma. Br Med J 2:685–686, 1976.

Maxwell, MH, Waks, AV, Schroth, PC, Karam, M, and Dornfeld, LP: Error in blood-pressure measurement due to incorrect cuff size in obese patients. Lancet I:33–36, 1982.

Julius, S, Ellis, CN, Pascual, AV, Matice, M, Hansson, L, Hunyor, SN, and Sandler, LN: Home blood pressure determination. Value in borderline ("labile") hypertension. JAMA 229:663–666, 1974.

2

PATHOGENESIS AND NATURAL HISTORY OF ESSENTIAL HYPERTENSION

The pathogenesis of essential hypertension is largely undefined, undoubtedly multifactorial, and highly complex, but some formulations have been proposed recently that appear to have merit. Regulation of the normal blood pressure itself is a complex process; although blood pressure is a function of cardiac output and peripheral resistance, each of these two major variables is influenced by multiple factors (Table 2–1). For example, cardiac output is affected by changes in extracellular fluid volume induced by alteration of sodium intake, renal function, and mineralocorticoid status. Changes in heart rate and contractility affect cardiac output more directly. Peripheral resistance is modulated in part by the sympathetic nervous system with its vasoconstrictor (alpha) and vasodilator (beta) components. Humoral influences on peripheral resistance are important and include angiotensin and catecholamines, which mediate vasoconstriction, and prostaglandins and kinins, which produce vasodilation. Finally, autoregulation may have a major effect on peripheral resistance, and it also serves as a link between cardiac output and peripheral resistance.

Autoregulation is the process by which changes in blood flow (cardiac output) produce alterations in peripheral resistance. When a primary increase in cardiac output occurs (and therefore an increase in mean blood pressure), there may be an initial decrease in peripheral resistance brought about by stretching of the arterioles and altered function of baroreceptors. After a while, however, the arterioles constrict in an autoregulatory fashion. Teleologically, this prevents excessive blood flow to peripheral tissues, but the mechanism remains undefined. Eventually, the increase in peripheral resistance may result in a return of cardiac output to its original level. The initial rise in blood pressure originally produced by the increase in cardiac output is now sustained by arteriolar vasoconstriction (Fig. 2–1).

Figure 2–2 depicts the so-called hypertensive mosaic. In essence, the mosaic provides a framework that emphasizes the interrelationship between the

TABLE 2–1. FACTORS INFLUENCING CARDIAC OUTPUT AND PERIPHERAL RESISTANCE

Cardiac Output	Peripheral Resistance

VIA EXTRACELLULAR FLUID VOLUME
  Salt
  Renal function
  Mineralocorticoids
	SYMPATHETIC NERVOUS SYSTEM
	  Vasoconstriction-alpha
	  Vasodilation-beta

HEART
  Pulse rate
  Contractility
	HUMORAL
	  Vasoconstriction-angiotensin,
	    catecholamines
	  Vasodilation-prostaglandins, kinins

	LOCAL Autoregulation

multiple factors modulating the blood pressure and the requirement to perfuse all tissues according to their needs. The various regulators are depicted around the circumference of the mosaic octagon and include humoral mediators such as angiotensin and catecholamines and the reactivity of the blood vessels and heart to humoral and neural stimulation. When all factors work in unison and equilibrium, a "normal" blood pressure is the result; a disturbance of the equilibrium may cause hypertension.

A suggested pathogenesis of essential hypertension, as summarized in Figure 2–3, stresses the importance of autoregulation and the evidence that suggests that excessive salt intake and the inability of the kidney (genetic predisposition?) to remove sodium effectively are crucial abnormalities in populations with a high incidence of essential hypertension. It should be emphasized, however, that the inability of the kidney to remove sodium effectively is assumed and is not clearly documented. Furthermore, if it occurs, it must be very early, because in established hypertension (without renal

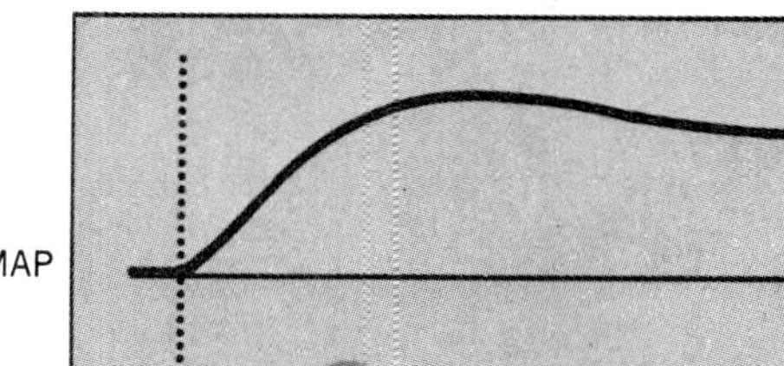

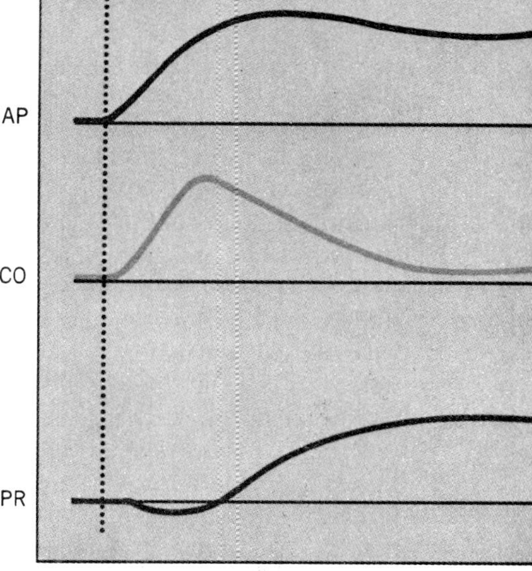

FIGURE 2–1. The hemodynamic alterations that occur as a result of a sustained increase in cardiac output. As can be seen, the initial rise in arterial pressure (MAP) occurs as a direct result of the increase in cardiac output (CO), and the total peripheral resistance (TPR) declines slightly. Subsequently, however, the increase in blood pressure is determined by the so-called autoregulatory increase in TPR. Thus, the hypertension induced by an increase in cardiac output, although initially attributable to an increment in blood flow, is maintained by an augmentation of TPR, cardiac output having returned to baseline. (Reproduced with permission from G. D. Searle & Co.: Clinician [Hypertension], 1973.)

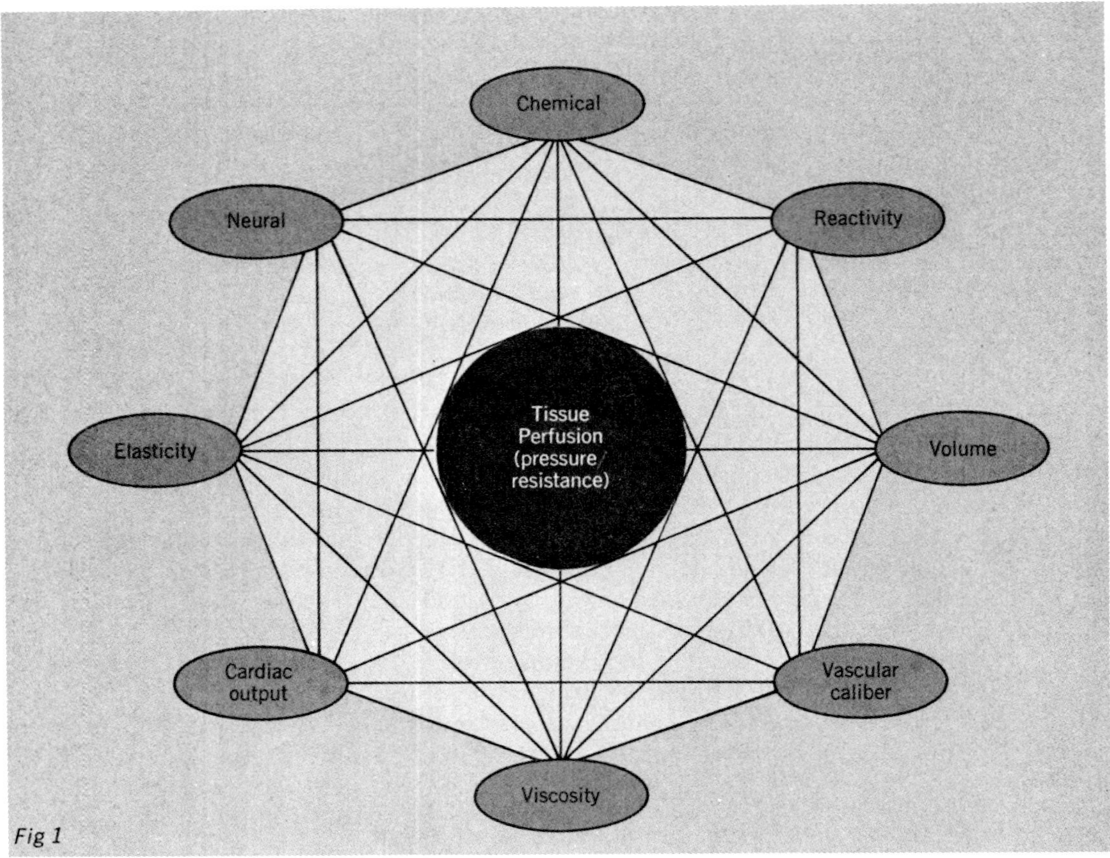

FIGURE 2–2. The hypertensive mosaic. This schema provides a framework that emphasizes the interrelationship between the multiple factors modulating the blood pressure and the requirement to perfuse all tissues according to their needs. When all factors work in unison and equilibrium, a "normal" blood pressure is the result; a disturbance of the equilibrium may cause hypertension. (Reproduced with permission from G. D. Searle & Co.: Clinician [Hypertension], 1973.)

failure), sodium loads are excreted in an exaggerated rather than an attenuated fashion.

Although the importance of the genetic contribution to essential hypertension is clear, the precise mechanism whereby such an abnormality exerts its pathophysiologic effects has not been elucidated. In Kaplan's schema, genetic predisposition plus excessive dietary sodium intake permits the renal retention of salt and water, which in turn leads to expansion of the extracellular fluid volume with resultant increased cardiac output. Autoregulation eventually causes vasoconstriction, and the patient ends up with a normal cardiac output and elevated total peripheral resistance. As can be seen in Figure 2–3, numerous other physiologic perturbations occur simultaneously, including the recently emphasized increase in vascular reactivity, which appears to result from increased sympathetic nervous system activity and abnormalities of the renin-angiotensin-aldosterone axis.

The natural history of essential hypertension can be related in part to the pathogenetic schema outlined above. Thus, humans destined to become hypertensive are influenced from a very early age by hereditary and environmental factors. Salt intake is almost surely one of the important variables influencing

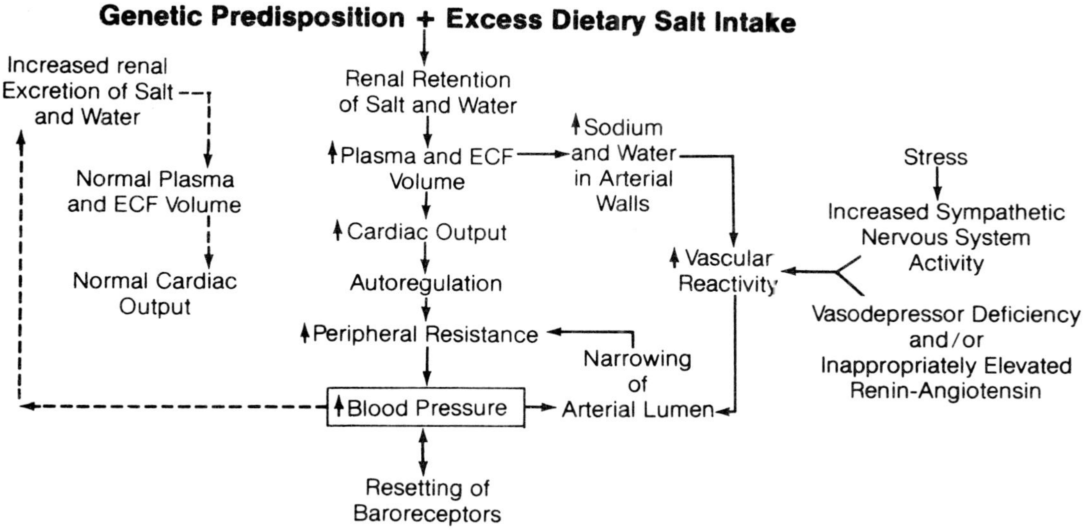

FIGURE 2–3. Schema for the possible pathogenesis of essential hypertension whereby multiple influences, including genetic predisposition, excess dietary salt intake, and adrenergic tone, may interact to produce hypertension. (Reproduced with permission from Kaplan, NM: Clinical Hypertension, 2nd ed. The Williams & Wilkins Co., Baltimore, 1978.)

the latter. In the so-called *prehypertensive* period (average age 10 to 30 years), cardiac output is increased while the blood pressure is normal or increased only on occasion (labile hypertension). Increased peripheral resistance and persistent hypertension characterize the largely asymptomatic period of *early hypertension*, which overlaps the first period and extends on the average until about age 40. In the prototypical case, the last 10-plus years of untreated *established* hypertension are characterized by the occurrence of any of the several complications.

Figure 2–4 depicts in a schematic fashion the natural history of untreated essential hypertension. Following the evolution from occasional into established

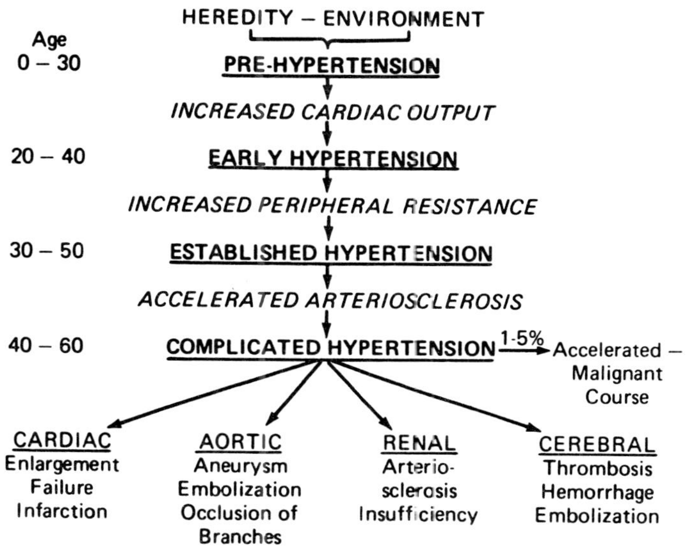

FIGURE 2–4. The natural history of untreated essential hypertension. Following the evolution from occasional into established hypertension, and after a long and variable asymptomatic period, a number of complications occur in various organs, including the heart, the kidney, and the central nervous system. (Reproduced with permission from Kaplan, NM: Clinical Hypertension, 3rd ed. The Williams & Wilkins Co., Baltimore, 1982.)

TABLE 2–2. POTENTIAL COMPLICATIONS OF HYPERTENSION

Related to Accelerated Arteriosclerosis	Target Organ	Related to Hypertension Per Se
Angina, myocardial infarction	Heart	Congestive heart failure
Occlusive phenomena	Arteries	Aortic dissection
Transient ischemic attacks, infarction	Brain	Cerebral hemorrhage, encephalopathy
Retinal vascular accidents, especially of occlusive type	Eye	Flame-shaped hemorrhages, exudates and papilledema
Renal vascular disease, sometimes exacerbating the degree of hypertension	Kidney	Arteriolar nephrosclerosis, sometimes with fibrinoid necrosis, renal insufficiency

hypertension and after a long and variable asymptomatic period, a number of complications occur in various organs, including the heart, the kidney, and the central nervous system.

Table 2–2 lists the potential complications of hypertension. These can be classified according to the target organ involved and as to whether they are related to accelerated arteriosclerosis or to hypertension per se. In the former group are included ischemic myocardial disease, peripheral vascular disease, stroke, retinal vascular accidents, and renal vascular disease. On the other hand, complications apparently caused by the increase in pressure per se include congestive heart failure, dissection of the aorta, cerebral hemorrhage, retinal hemorrhages and exudates, and arteriolar nephrosclerosis.

Recent data suggest that isolated elevation of systolic pressure, which is particularly common in the elderly, may be just as hazardous as increased levels of diastolic blood pressure in producing the various hypertensive complications (see Chapter 11).

PROMINENT COMPLICATIONS OF HYPERTENSION

The following section will consider in greater detail the most prominent complications of hypertension, i.e., those affecting the heart, the kidneys, and the central nervous system.

Hypertension and the Heart

Of note, recent data suggest the importance of the active role that the heart plays in the pathophysiology of hypertension (in addition to the damage suffered by that organ as a result of persistent hypertension). Although the precise factors that modulate the increased cardiac output that characterizes *early* hypertension are unknown, certain factors appear to be incriminated, including cardiopulmonary redistribution of blood volume, primary overactivity of the sympathetic nervous system and, perhaps in some circumstances, systemic vasoconstriction resulting from reflexes induced by myocardial ischemia.

As discussed nicely in a recent editorial in the Lancet (1983), the implications of cardiac hypertrophy for the hypertensive patient are far from well understood. In animals, hypertrophy develops soon after the onset of experimentally induced hypertension. That activation of the sympathetic nervous system may be a necessary factor in the development of left ventricular hypertrophy is suggested by its obviation by methyldopa but not by hydralazine.

Although late in the hypertensive process the structural damage that attends chronic left ventricular hypertrophy is obviously harmful, it is generally agreed that before this time it is beneficial in terms of sustaining cardiac output. On the other hand, if antihypertensive therapy reduces hypertrophy to a greater degree than blood pressure, or diminishes coronary blood flow reserve by lowering blood pressure without reducing hypertrophy, problems might arise. Since it appears that antihypertensive agents may have quite variable effects on cardiac hypertrophy, prospective studies need to be done to sort out these problems.

Hypertension and the Central Nervous System

The central nervous system is a major target organ for the expression of hypertensive disease. The disease may appear as a stroke in patients with localized vascular damage or as encephalopathy in those exposed to exceedingly high levels of blood pressure. Conversely, successful control of the blood pressure is rewarded by a marked reduction in the risk of CNS complications.

Hypertension is the major cause of cerebrovascular disease. In the Framingham study, the degree of risk was shown to increase progressively with the age and level of blood pressure. Both systolic and diastolic hypertension are detrimental. At diastolic levels greater than 100 mm Hg, the increase in the incidence of stroke is proportionately greater than that for coronary artery disease. Similarly, isolated systolic hypertension is associated with a much greater incidence of strokes than that observed in normotensive people of the same age. Figure 2–5 illustrates the relationship between the level of systolic blood pressure and the occurrence of strokes, heart attacks, and peripheral vascular disease as determined by the Framingham study. As can be seen, the risk of developing a thrombotic stroke is approximately four times normal when the systolic pressure has increased two standard deviations above the normal average.

Cerebrovascular disease in the hypertensive patient assumes a wide array of forms. Some are seen only in the setting of hypertension, including hypertensive hemorrhage, hypertensive encephalopathy, and lacunar-type infarctions. Other types of cerebrovascular disease, such as emboli, massive infarction, and transient ischemic attacks, have a multifactorial pathogenesis but are observed more frequently in the presence of hypertension.

Hypertensive Encephalopathy. Hypertensive encephalopathy is the subacute onset of altered consciousness, progressing from drowsiness to stupor to coma and accompanied by headaches, nausea, vomiting, visual blurring, and transient neurologic disturbances, including seizures. Untreated, this is a disastrous condition, often resulting in demise within several hours to a few days.

Unfortunately, not every hypertensive patient with altered mental status has hypertensive encephalopathy. The differential diagnosis is long, and the clinician must remember that many primary intracranial processes, particularly those that exert a mass effect, may increase the blood pressure markedly. In such patients, the blood pressure may be highly sensitive to antihypertensive agents, and care must be taken to avoid frank hypotension. Rarely, posterior

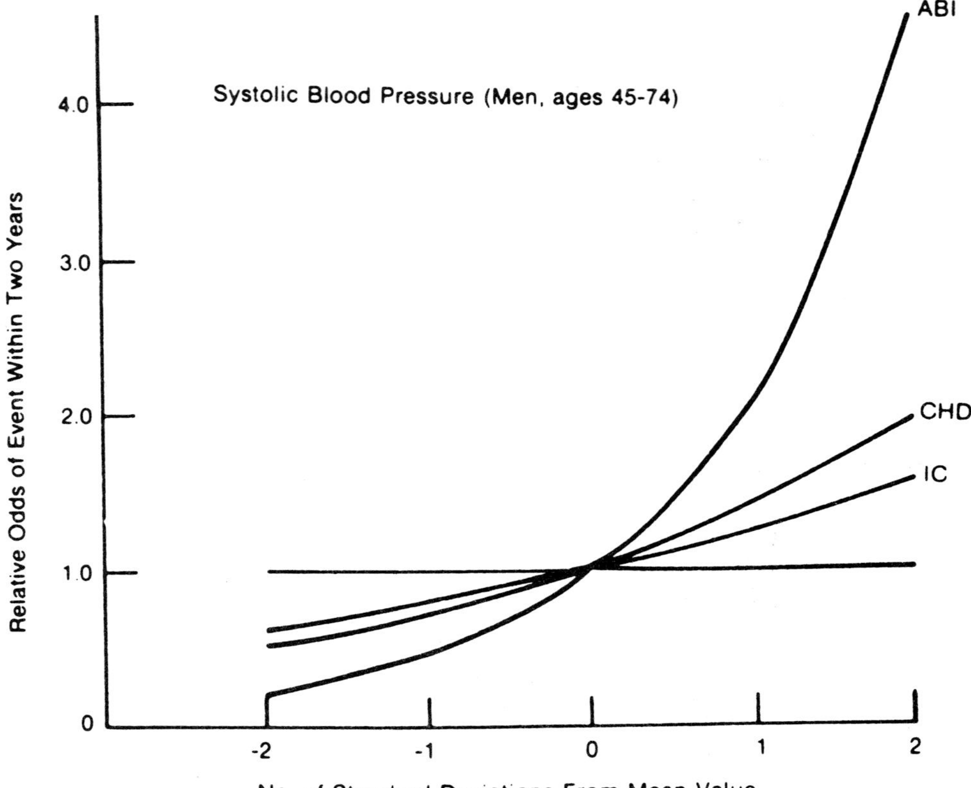

FIGURE 2–5. The relationship between the level of systolic blood pressure and the occurrence of strokes (atherothrombotic brain infarction, *ABI*), heart attacks (coronary heart disease, *CHD*), and peripheral vascular disease (intermittent claudication, *IC*) as determined by the Framingham study. As can be seen, the risk of developing a thrombotic stroke is approximately four times normal when the systolic pressure has increased two standard deviations above the normal average. (Reproduced with permission from Gordon, T, and Kannel, WB: J.A.M.A. *221*:663, Aug. 14, 1972. Copyright 1972, American Medical Association.)

fossa lesions, such as hemangioblastoma, may even induce a syndrome mimicking pheochromocytoma. Thus, sometimes the diagnosis of hypertensive encephalopathy must be in part retrospective, since the diagnosis is strongly supported by a prompt and marked clinical improvement when the blood pressure is lowered.

Although the pathophysiology of hypertensive encephalopathy remains controversial, a widely accepted postulate to account for the production of the cerebral edema that characterizes this condition is a so-called breakthrough of cerebral autoregulation. This means that in the face of extreme hypertension, the intracerebral vessels become unable to constrict (and may even dilate), leading to marked overperfusion of the brain. This concept is essentially the opposite of the time-honored theory that excessive vasoconstriction results in cerebral edema secondary to profound ischemia. Perhaps both phenomena occur either coterminously or sequentially in varying areas of the brain.

Hypertensive Retinopathy. Retinal vascular changes occur in all forms of hypertension—mild, moderate, and accelerated. Examination of the fundus is an excellent way for clinicians to assess the particular stage of the disease.

Constriction is the normal retinal response to a rise in blood pressure, thereby raising resistance, which keeps the blood flow to tissues constant. In hypertension, therefore, as long as this autoregulation is intact, changes may occur in the vessel wall, but there will be no retinopathy. In analogy with the changes in the cerebral circulation, the appearance of hemorrhages and exudates seems to reflect a breakdown in the autoregulatory response.

Hypertension and the Kidney

The kidney is one of the major organs that is damaged as a result of long-standing elevation in blood pressure. Arteriolar nephrosclerosis is the descriptive term applied to the pathologic changes produced in the kidney. Of course, hypertension may also accelerate atherosclerotic changes that occur independently in the major arteries of the kidney. On the other hand, malignant hypertension, with its characteristic fibrinoid necrosis, may be superimposed on arteriolar nephrosclerosis. Finally, the adverse renal effects of hypertension may act coterminously, and often with devastating effect, with those of other renal diseases, particularly chronic glomerulonephritis and diabetic nephrosclerosis.

Hypertensive renal disease is a major cause of impaired renal function in the United States, particularly in patient populations deriving from inner city areas or containing a high percentage of blacks. Renal insufficiency is a late complication of essential hypertension, occurring after several years. Its progress tends to be relatively slow, and unless blood pressure is controlled, inexorable.

Although not yet conclusively established by large-scale controlled studies, a diverse body of data has been accruing over the last several years that lends considerable support to the premise that the renal lesions of *accelerated* or *malignant hypertension* are blunted and in some cases reversed if good blood pressure control is initiated before terminal renal failure. In fact, as will be emphasized in the therapeutic section of this book (see Chapter 6) and in the case studies, developing renal failure should serve as a red flag to the clinician to begin therapy immediately. Initially, therapy may result in a further decrement in renal function. Nevertheless, it is crucial to maintain blood pressure control. This frequently leads after several days to several weeks or more to improvement in glomerular filtration rate (GFR). Indeed, there have been several reports (and we have seen examples) of patients whose renal function has improved after several months of hemodialytic therapy. On the other hand, if hypertension is allowed to persist uncontrolled, eventual severe irreversible renal failure is almost inevitable.

Unfortunately, the data regarding the beneficial effect of antihypertensive therapy in preventing or reversing the renal failure of *chronic essential hypertension without acceleration* are not at hand. Theoretically, in this circumstance, as opposed to the above situation in malignant hypertension, once renal failure has occurred the kidneys are usually already small, implying marked nephron loss, fibrosis, and limited reversibility.

Hypertensive Crisis

A true *hypertensive crisis* occurs in far fewer than one per cent of all patients with essential hypertension. These situations are characterized by extremely high levels of blood pressure (usually but not always, diastolic pressure exceeds 130 mm Hg) and by evidence of potentially life-threatening end-organ dysfunction. In general, the pressure should be reduced within minutes to a few days in order to reduce the risk of serious or fatal complications. Table 2–3 lists the clinical conditions justifiably termed hypertensive crisis. It is just as

TABLE 2–3. HYPERTENSIVE CRISIS

Crisis	*Not Crisis*
Hypertensive encephalopathy	Asymptomatic marked hypertension without severe acute end-organ dysfunction
Extreme hypertension with acute pulmonary edema	Hypertension with minimal evidence of congestive heart failure
Extreme hypertension with acute aortic dissection	Hypertension and evidence of a thrombotic stroke
Extreme hypertension with intracerebral hemorrhage	
Extreme hypertension with an acute myocardial infarction	
Malignant hypertension	

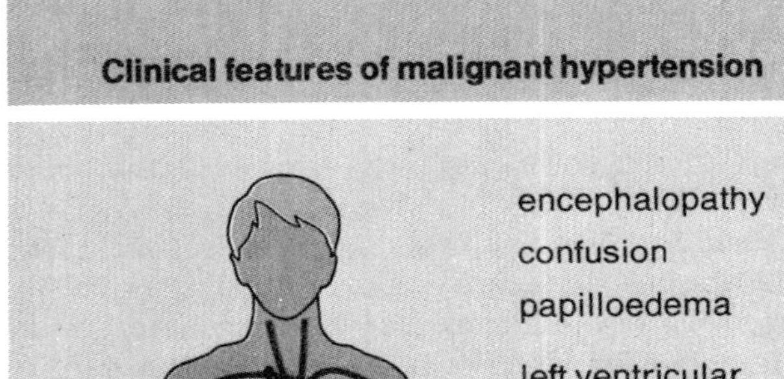

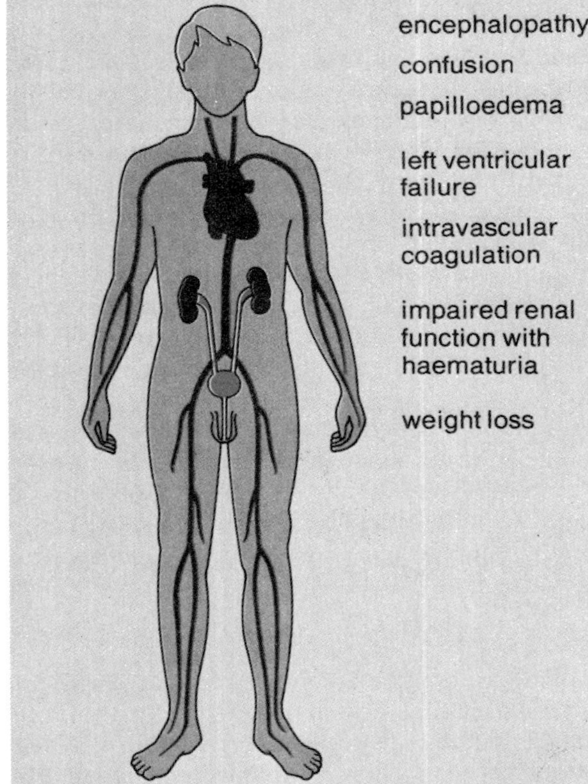

FIGURE 2–6. The clinical features of malignant hypertension. Although patients with malignant hypertension may initially remain asymptomatic, the condition is typically associated with florid clinical features representing the clinical correlates of end-organ damage. (Reproduced from Hypertension Illustrated by WS Peart, PS Sever, JD Swales and R Tarazi, courtesy of Gower Medical Publishing.)

important for the physician to be aware of what is *not* a true crisis (Table 2–3) as to know what *is*, since submitting a patient to the risk of highly aggressive therapy in the former situation represents an unwarranted hazard. As can be seen in the table, a very high pressure, for example 200/140 mm Hg, without evidence of acute, severe, end-organ dysfunction, is a serious medical problem but not a hypertensive emergency.

Malignant hypertension is a clinical entity that may or may not be associated with other types of hypertensive crisis such as hypertensive encephalopathy. Figure 2–6 illustrates the clinical features of malignant hypertension. Although patients with malignant hypertension may initially remain asymptomatic, the condition is typically associated with florid clinical features representing the clinical correlates of end-organ damage. By definition, a patient with malignant hypertension has retinal papilledema, almost always together with flame-shaped hemorrhages and exudates. Pathologically, this condition is characterized by fibrinoid necrosis of arterioles, particularly those of the kidney. If treatment is not successful, the incidence of fatal complications, including rapidly developing renal failure, is extraordinarily high, and more than 90 per cent of patients will be dead within a 1-to-2–year period.

REFERENCES

Berglund, G, Andersson, O, and Wilhelmsen, L: Prevalence of primary and secondary hypertension: Studies in a random population sample. Br Med J 2:554–556, 1976.

Brown, JJ, Lever, AF, Robertson, JIS, and Schalekamp, MA: Pathogenesis of essential hypertension. Lancet I:1217–1219, 1976.

Editorial: Genetics, environment, and hypertension. Lancet I:681–682, 1983.

Hollenberg, NK, Williams, GH, and Adams, DF: Essential hypertension: abnormal renal vascular and endocrine responses to a mild psychological stimulus. Hypertension 3:11–17, 1981.

Lund-Johansen, P: Haemodynamics in essential hypertension. Clin Sci Molec Med 59:343S–354S, 1980.

Hollenberg, NK: Renal perfusion and vascular reactivity in essential hypertension. *In* Laragh, JH, Buhler, FR, and Seldin, DW (eds.): Frontiers in Hypertension Research. Springer-Verlag, New York, 1981.

Haber, E: The renin-angiotensin system and hypertension. Kidney Int 15:427–444, 1979.

Case, DB, Wallace, JN, Keim, HJ, Weber, MA, Sealy, JE, and Laragh, JH: Possible role of renin in hypertension as suggested by renin-sodium profiling and inhibition of converting enzyme. N Engl J Med 296:641–646, 1977.

Kaplan, NM: The prognostic implications of plasma renin in essential hypertension. JAMA 231:167–170, 1975.

Atlas, SA, and Case, DB: Renin in essential hypertension. Clin Endocrinol Metab 10:537–575, 1981.

Dunn, MJ, and Tannen, RL: Low-renin hypertension. Kidney Int 5:317–325, 1974.

Kesteloot, H, and Geboers, J: Calcium and blood pressure. Lancet I:813–815, 1982.

Freestone, S, and Ramsay, LE: Pressor effect of coffee and cigarette smoking in hypertensive patients. Clin Sci 63:403S–405S, 1982.

Friedman, GDI, Klatsky, AL, and Siegelaub, AB: Alcohol, tobacco, and hypertension. Hypertension 4(Suppl. III):143–150, 1982.

Bechgaard, P: A 40 years' followup study of 1000 untreated hypertensive subjects. Clin Sci Molec Med 51:673S–675S, 1976.

Perera, G: Hypertensive vascular disease; description and natural history. J Chronic Dis 1:33–42, 1955.

Veterans Administration Cooperative Study Group on Antihypertensive Agents: Effects of treatment on morbidity in hypertension. Results in patients with diastolic blood pressures averaging 115 through 129 mm Hg. JAMA 202:116–122, 1967.

Veterans Administration Cooperative Study Group on Antihypertensive Agents: Effects of treatment on morbidity in hypertension. II. Results in patients with diastolic blood pressure averaging 90 through 114 mm Hg. JAMA 213:1143–1152, 1970.

Culpepper, WS, III, Sodt, PC, Messerli, FH, Rusckhaupt, DG, and Arcilla, RA: Cardiac status in juvenile borderline hypertension. Ann Intern Med 98:1–7, 1983.

Editorial: The heart and hypertension. Lancet I:165–166, 1983.

Tarazi, RC: The role of the heart in hypertension. Clin Sci Molec Med 63:3475–3585, 1982.

Tarazi, RC, Ibrahim, MM, Dustan, HP, and Ferrario, CM: Cardiac factors in hypertension. Circ Res 34: (Suppl I):213–221, 1974.

Kannel, WB, McGee, D, and Gordon, T: A general cardiovascular risk profile: The Framingham study. Am J Cardiol 38:46–51, 1976.

Guyton, AC, Coleman, TG, Cowley, AW, Jr, Scheel, KW, Manning, RD, Jr, and Norman, RA: Arterial pressure regulation: Overriding dominance of the kidneys in long-term regulation and in hypertension. Am J Med 52:584–594, 1972.

Ferris, TF: The kidney and hypertension. Arch Intern Med 142:1889–1895, 1982.

Kaplan, NM (guest ed.): Hypertension and the kidney. Seminars in Nephrology 3:1–72, 1983.

3

SECONDARY HYPERTENSION

The overwhelming majority of hypertensive patients have *essential* hypertension; only a relatively small subgroup (varying according to several studies from 2 to 10 per cent) have *secondary* hypertension. The reader will readily observe that more attention has been devoted to a discussion of secondary forms of hypertension than to essential hypertension. It should be emphasized that this obviously does not connote a lack of importance of essential hypertension; rather, it reflects the clinical orientation of this book. Thus, we have minimized discussion of the vast speculative literature regarding the factors underlying essential hypertension.

The most common secondary causes of chronic hypertension are summarized in Table 3–1. It should be emphasized that the headings in Table 3–1 subtend several subgroups; i.e., renal parenchymal disease includes a number of specific disease entities, including pyelonephritis, glomerulonephritis, hypoplastic kidneys, and polycystic kidney disease. Similarly, aldosteronism is not a single entity but includes patients with a single adrenal cortical adenoma and bilateral nodular cortical hyperplasia, as well as atypical forms such as glucocorticoid-sensitive aldosteronism. The more clinically important of these entities will be discussed briefly.

We have already emphasized that the clinician should not evaluate every hypertensive patient for a secondary cause; rather, he must be able to exercise clinical judgment in the selection of those patients who ultimately will undergo a diagnostic evaluation. Figure 3–1 summarizes in schematic fashion the major historical and physical findings that suggest the likelihood of secondary hypertension.

THE RENIN-ANGIOTENSIN SYSTEM IN HYPERTENSION

Even though the precise role of the renin-angiotensin system in the pathogenesis of hypertension is controversial, measurements of plasma renin are useful in the diagnosis of correctable hypertension secondary to a number of disease entities, including renal artery stenosis and hyperaldosteronism. Furthermore, although the topic is controversial, several authors have proposed that it may be important to categorize essential hypertensive patients into low renin, normal renin, and high renin subgroups, and that the subsequent choice

TABLE 3–1. CAUSES OF SECONDARY HYPERTENSION

A. RENAL
   1. Glomerulonephritis
   2. Pyelonephritis
   3. Obstructive uropathy
   4. Collagen diseases
   5. Congenital disorders
   6. Diabetes mellitus
   7. Hypersensitivity angiitis
   8. Renal tumors (particularly hemangiopericytoma)

B. ADRENAL
   1. Primary aldosteronism
   2. Pheochromocytoma
   3. Cushing's syndrome
   4. Adrenogenital syndromes

C. CENTRAL NERVOUS SYSTEM
   1. Brain tumor
   2. Increased intracranial pressure from any cause (particularly from posterior fossa lesions)
   3. Guillain-Barré syndrome
   4. Bulbar poliomyelitis

D. VASCULAR
   1. Renal artery stenosis
   2. Coarctation of the aorta

E. OTHER
   1. Psychogenic
   2. Drug-induced (oral contraceptives, licorice, sympathomimetic medications, including nose drops and anorectics)
   3. Eclampsia
   4. Polycythemia
   5. Hypothyroidism
   6. Acromegaly
   7. Hypercalcemia

of the optimal agent for the treatment of hypertension is facilitated by knowledge of the renin status of the patient. Therefore, it seems appropriate to begin this discussion of secondary hypertension with a consideration of the renin-angiotensin system.

Physiology of the Renin-Angiotensin System

The components and physiology of the renin-angiotensin-aldosterone system are shown in Figure 3–2. The enzyme renin is formed and stored principally in the juxtaglomerular apparatus of the kidney, from which it is released into both renal venous blood and renal lymph. The substrate for renin, angiotensinogen, is an alpha$_2$ globulin synthesized by the liver. Renin reacts in the plasma with angiotensinogen, splitting off an inactive decapeptide, angiotensin I. Angiotensin I is hydrolyzed within the circulation by a converting enzyme into an octapeptide, angiotensin II, which is largely responsible for the several physiologic and pathophysiologic effects of the renin-angiotensin system.

Measurement of Components of the Renin-Angiotensin System

Since renin itself cannot be measured directly, evaluation of the activity of the renin-angiotensin system under both normal and pathologic conditions usually entails assessment by measurement of other components of the system.

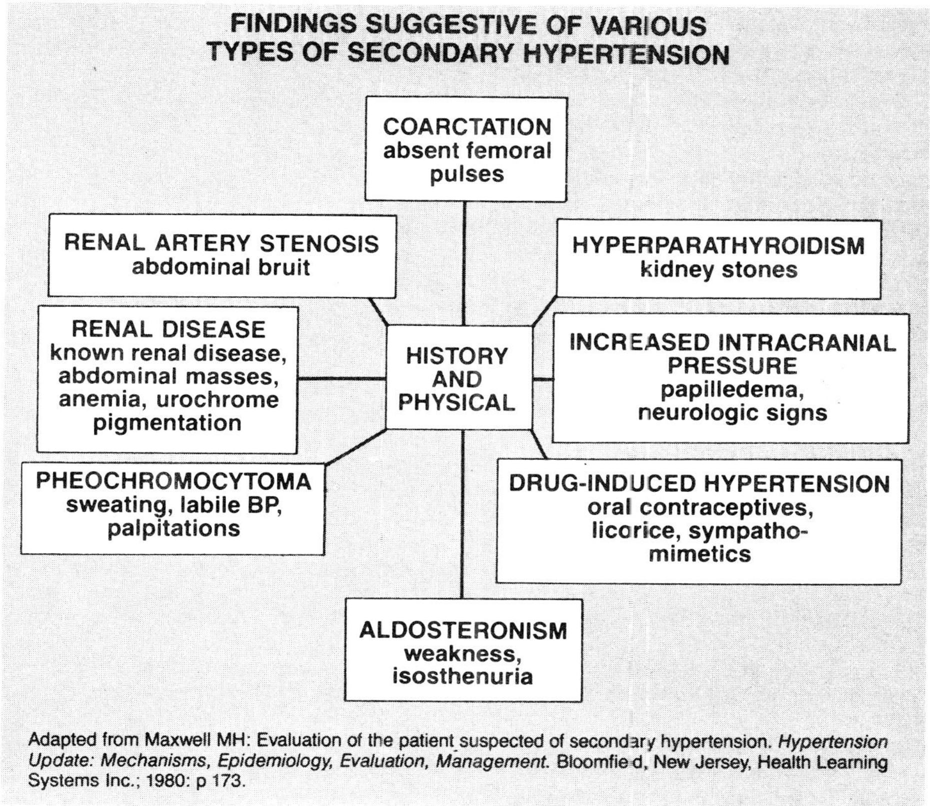

FIGURE 3–1. Summary of the major historical and physical findings that suggest the likelihood of secondary hypertension. (Reproduced with permission from "Pretreatment Evaluation of the Patient with Hypertension," from the program *Dialogues in Hypertension*. Vol. 4, No. 5, September 1982, p. 3. James C. Hunt, M.D., Executive Editor. Copyright 1982 by Health Learning Systems, Inc., Bloomfield, N.J.)

The amount of angiotensin I generated in the reaction between renin and angiotensinogen under defined conditions (temperature, pH, substrate concentration, and incubation time) is determined by radioimmunoassay. Methods that do not add substrate in excess determine *plasma renin activity* (PRA), a *rate* measurement.

Although radioimmunoassays for angiotensin II were developed first, measurement of angiotensin I has found wider applicability in clinical medicine because plasma samples can be used directly in the angiotensin I radioimmunoassay without prior extraction procedures. Of the various means described for assessing the activity of the renin-angiotensin system, measurement of plasma renin activity is most widely used. Although the availability of commercially prepackaged kits suggests that this determination is within the capability of most radioisotope laboratories, the clinician should be somewhat leery. Considerable care must be exercised in the performance of the assay, which presents methodologic pitfalls of greater complexity than those found in many other commonly used radioimmunoassays. Furthermore, as will be evident from subsequent considerations, even accurately performed renin measurements can be interpreted only if samples are obtained under clinically defined circumstances. Random, single determinations are often meaningless.

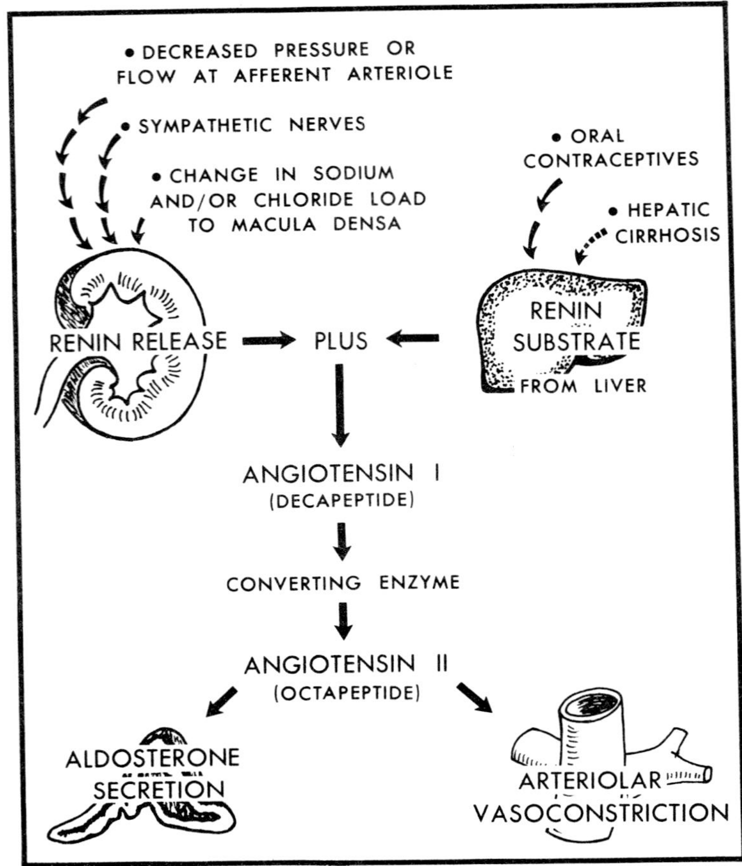

FIGURE 3–2. Overview of the components and physiology of the renin-angiotensin-aldosterone system. At the time of acute circulatory impairment, activation of the renin-angiotensin-aldosterone system results in the conservation of sodium (and thereby ECF) and maintenance of blood pressure with restoration of circulatory homeostasis. (From Epstein, M, and Oster, J. *In* Halsted, JA, and Halsted, CH: The Laboratory in Clinical Medicine, 2nd ed. W. B. Saunders Co., Philadelphia, 1981.)

Factors Influencing Circulating Renin and Angiotensin Levels

As shown in Table 3–2, sodium balance is a major determinant of renin-angiotensin activity; sodium deprivation leads to an increase in PRA, whereas high dietary sodium intake depresses PRA. Potassium loading exerts an inhibiting effect on the renin-angiotensin system, but this effect appears to be relatively minor and is readily overwhelmed by the effects of changes in sodium balance. Ambulation and the upright posture lead to an increase in PRA.

A variety of medications have been shown to exert important effects on renin release. Diuretic agents and vasodilators stimulate renin release, but most beta-receptor blocking agents, methyldopa, clonidine, and perhaps prazosin suppress renin, at least transiently.

Sampling Conditions for PRA

Blood is collected in Na-EDTA–containing vacuum tubes (such as Vacutainers), and the time of collection and previous activity of the subject are noted. The sample must be mixed immediately with the anticoagulant by repeated gentle inversion of the tube and chilled until separation. After centrifugation at 4° C, the plasma is separated and stored in the frozen state until ready for measurement. Since PRA varies markedly with changes in sodium balance, it is of value to relate the determinations of PRA to the concurrent 24-hour urinary sodium excretion. Although it was perhaps an overstatement to assert

TABLE 3–2. FACTORS INFLUENCING CIRCULATING LEVELS OF RENIN AND ANGIOTENSIN

1. Sodium balance
2. Potassium balance
3. Posture and activity
4. Circadian rhythm
5. Menstrual cycle (higher in the luteal phase)
6. Drugs
   a. *Those that stimulate renin*
      (1) Benzothiadiazine-type diuretics (thiazides)
      (2) Spironolactone
      (3) Diazoxide
   b. *Those that suppress renin*
      (1) Beta-receptor blocking agents
      (2) Methyldopa
      (3) Clonidine (at least transiently)
      (4) Prazosin ?
      (5) Licorice (glycyrrhizinic acid component)
   c. *Variable effects on angiotensin II*
      (1) Estrogen-progestogen–type oral contraceptives

Modified from Epstein, M. The Kidney 10:1–6, Jan. 1977.

that random samples are valueless, the importance of standardizing as many dietary and activity conditions as possible when collecting blood samples for PRA is clear.

RENOVASCULAR HYPERTENSION

Renovascular hypertension (RVHT) is thought by many to comprise the most common cause of curable secondary hypertension. Renovascular hypertension refers to hypertension caused by renal ischemia. Several lines of evidence have suggested strongly that increased renin secretion is responsible for the initial generation of this type of hypertension.

The myriad of anatomic abnormalities other than simple renal artery stenosis that can result in renovascular hypertension are listed in Table 3–3.

TABLE 3–3. CAUSES OF RENOVASCULAR HYPERTENSION

1. Atherosclerosis
2. Fibromuscular dysplasia
3. Miscellaneous arterial abnormalities
   a. Aortic coarctation
   b. Embolic renal artery occlusion
   c. Aneurysm of the renal artery
   d. Arteriovenous malformation
   e. Diffuse arteritis
   f. Perirenal or periarterial fibrosis
4. Diffuse bilateral renal ischemia
   a. Accelerated hypertension
   b. Necrotizing vasculitis
   c. Hepatitis-B antigenemia
   d. Intravenous drug abuse
5. Renal artery stenosis following renal transplantation

These lesions may involve the main renal artery on one or both sides, accessory renal arteries, and extrarenal and intrarenal segmental branches.

Prevalence of Renovascular Hypertension

Since secondary hypertension is not (and should not) be routinely excluded in all newly discovered hypertensive patients, the true prevalence of renovascular hypertension is not known. The published figures from large referral centers probably overestimate the frequency, because renal arteriography is often ordered only in patients who are to a considerable degree preselected.

Thus, in a large series of 1070 patients referred to Vanderbilt University Hospital, 16 per cent had physiologically important renal artery stenosis. The incidence was even higher in white patients with accelerated hypertension. Conversely, of approximately 26,000 patients with hypertension who were evaluated between 1973 and 1975 at the Mayo Clinic, less than 100 (0.4 per cent) had proven renovascular hypertension. Although the true prevalence of RVHT probably lies somewhere between these values, it is almost surely much closer to the Mayo Clinic than the Vanderbilt figure. In addition to the severity of the patient's hypertension, the incidence varies according to the ethnic composition, the age of the population studied, and the criteria used in the selection of patients for study and for establishing the diagnosis.

There is still controversy over which hypertensive subjects merit a work-up for renovascular hypertension. In general, the emphasis recently has swung away from extensive work-ups in every patient with recently recognized hypertension and toward early initiation of effective pharmacologic therapy. Nevertheless, there are some generally accepted criteria concerning whom to evaluate. These include patients with the following:

1. Recent onset of moderate to severe hypertension.
2. Sudden unexplained exacerbation of preexisting hypertension.
3. Hypertension associated with the finding of an abdominal bruit.
4. Hypertension developing subsequent to abdominal trauma.
5. Onset of hypertension at an age atypical for essential hypertension (less than 25 to 30 years), particularly if there is no family history.
6. Severe hypertension resistant to appropriate pharmacologic management.
7. Unusually marked decrement of renal function following initiation of drug therapy for hypertension.

If one decides that a patient's findings definitely warrant a work-up for renovascular hypertension, the work-up should be complete and pushed to its logical conclusion, i.e., renal arteriogram (or digital video subtraction angiography) and bilateral renal vein PRA determinations (see pp. 29–30).

Equally important is the knowledge of who should not be evaluated for renovascular hypertension. In addition to all patients not fulfilling the above-mentioned criteria one must abide by the general rule not to work up patients for any condition if therapy is not to depend upon the results of the evaluation. Thus, since most investigators agree that the older patient (age exceeding 50 years), the patient with important vascular disease in other arterial beds (i.e., cerebral, coronary, or peripheral circulations), and the patient with a major degree of renal insufficiency (serum creatinine levels greater than 2.0 to 2.5 mg/dl) frequently do not benefit from surgery, they should not be worked up. This viewpoint may require reassessment in the light of the advent of transluminal angioplasty (see Chapter 14).

In evaluating the patient with suspected renovascular hypertension, it should be appreciated that renovascular disease (narrowing of the renal arterial tree) is not synonymous with renovascular hypertension. Since numerous studies have demonstrated that patients with renal artery stenosis are more frequently normotensive than hypertensive, the presence of a stenotic lesion is often merely an incidental finding. *It is incumbent upon the clinician to demonstrate that the vascular lesion in his hypertensive patient is hemodynamically significant and causally related to the hypertension.* Only then can one anticipate confidently the relief of hypertension by revascularization, angioplasty, or nephrectomy.

Clinical attempts to distinguish the patient with renovascular hypertension from the patient with essential hypertension are difficult. Recent studies of patients with essential hypertension and carefully matched patients with surgically cured renovascular disease have disclosed only minor differences in the clinical characteristics of these two groups. The only feature that was of clear discriminatory value was the presence of an abdominal bruit (12 per cent incidence in renovascular hypertension vs. only 1 per cent in patients with essential hypertension). One of the most readily available tests to the clinician is the examination for an abdominal bruit. It should be emphasized that bruits present only in systole are of little value, since they are frequently found in patients with essential hypertension and in normal subjects. In contrast, a number of investigators have stressed the specific value of an abdominal bruit with both a systolic and a diastolic component. It has been suggested that systolic-diastolic bruits may be identified in 40 to 60 per cent of patients with surgically responsive renovascular hypertension.

Renal Artery Bruits

Despite the diagnostic importance of renal artery bruits, these often hard to hear murmurs are often missed, in part because of poor technique. The following recommendation of Grim is well advised.

The examination should be carried out in a quiet room; background noise, as from fans or television, may make the bruits impossible to discern. The physician's concentration must be intent. A bruit with both systolic and diastolic components is the key finding. The patient should lie supine with the knees flexed. The stethoscope is placed lightly on the epigastrium. The quality and pitch of the diastolic component of the bruit is very similar to that of a soft aortic insufficiency murmur. If the above procedure is negative, pressure is then exerted on the head of the stethoscope, which is pushed down over the aorta. If nothing is heard in the center of the epigastrium, the head of the stethoscope is moved in all directions. Firm pressure may be necessary; it is very difficult to cause a bruit with a diastolic component by pushing too hard.

Since the history, physical examination and routine laboratory studies may not be helpful in identifying patients who deserve a work-up for renovascular hypertension, a number of tests have been proposed (Table 3–4).

The appropriate sequence of tests for establishing the diagnosis of renovascular hypertension is controversial. Screening tests such as a rapid-sequence intravenous pyelogram (IVP) (also referred to as a urogram) or renogram may suggest that renovascular hypertension is present, but many clinicians perform renal angiography as the initial examination. Selective renal angiography permits the anatomic delineation of a renal arterial lesion such as unilateral stenosis of the main renal artery or occlusive disease of the smaller arteries (second-, third-, and occasionally fourth-order vessels).

TABLE 3–4. TESTS USEFUL IN THE EVALUATION OF CURABLE RENOVASCULAR HYPERTENSION

I. SCREENING PROCEDURES
  A. Rapid sequence intravenous pyelogram (IVP)
  B. Radioisotope renogram—may be substituted for IVP when performed accurately
II. CONFIRMATORY PROCEDURES
  A. Renal vein PRA levels—to be determined in patients with abnormal IVP compatible with renal ischemia or when clinical suspicion of renovascular hypertension is high
  B. Renal arteriography (if renal venous PRA ratio > 1.5)
  C. In selected cases, consider administration of an angiotensin antagonist such as saralasin or converting enzyme inhibitor

A number of studies have indicated that the rapid-sequence IVP constitutes the single most important screening test for renovascular hypertension. The Cooperative Study of Renovascular Hypertension has shown that such IVP's are abnormal in 78 per cent of the patients with renovascular hypertension and in only 11 per cent of hypertensive patients with normal arteriograms (i.e., "false positives"). These results may not be entirely representative, however, since they were obtained from a selected population (many patients were referred specifically because they had abnormal urograms). Nevertheless, the low number of false positives, the low complication rate, and the general availability of the procedure serve to make the urogram the most useful initial screening test in the evaluation of hypertensive patients suspected of having renovascular hypertension.

The renogram has also been advocated as a screening test for renovascular hypertension, but its utility overlaps to a great extent with that of the rapid-sequence IVP. We do not utilize the renogram as a screening procedure except in specific instances when a rapid-sequence IVP is contraindicated (history of reaction to radiocontrast dye, advanced age, etc.).

Digital Video Subtraction Angiography

The high cost and morbidity associated with selection of operative candidates for surgical cure has tended to bridle the enthusiasm for screening for renovascular hypertension. Recent reports of the success of digital video subtraction angiography (DVSA) have suggested an alternative diagnostic approach. In brief, DVSA requires only an intravenous contrast injection to display the abdominal aorta and its branches. Its proponents claim that it is relatively safe, easy, and inexpensive, requires neither sedation nor hospitalization either beforehand or afterward, and gives reliable information concerning renal artery stenosis. Hillman et al. have compared the average cost for performing DVSA at their institution with the conventional protocol comprising excretory urography, radionuclide studies, and arteriography and have found savings that approached 75 per cent.

Although PRA values obtained in the upright position have been advocated as an additional screening test for renovascular hypertension, the majority of studies indicate that peripheral PRA is a screening test of limited usefulness for renovascular hypertension unless it is elevated above the 95th percentile of values found in patients with essential hypertension. Thus, Grim et al. have suggested that a 2-hr upright PRA value may be helpful if it exceeds 30 ng/ml/

3 hr (normal is 7.1 ± 0.3 ng/ml/3 hr; 95 per cent of patients had values <15 ng/ml/3 hr). Under these circumstances, the test has a sensitivity of only 27 per cent; however, the specificity is 95 per cent. In this regard, the recent report of Grim et al. is of interest. These investigators noted that the screening combination of IVP, systolic-diastolic abdominal bruit, and upright PRA determination yielded a test sensitivity of 93 per cent with a specificity of 92 per cent. The authors concluded that if one or more of the three tests are abnormal, further work-up (arteriogram, renal vein PRA, etc.) should be strongly considered.

Saralasin Diagnostic Test

Saralasin is a polypeptide analogue of angiotensin II that competes for angiotensin II receptors in blood vessels and other tissues and blocks the pressure response to exogenous angiotensin I and angiotensin II in a dose-dependent fashion. It is proposed as a diagnostic tool both to identify patients with renovascular hypertension and to predict the outcome of surgery.

The premise of this test is that in a patient with a "high renin" type of hypertension, the administration of saralasin will cause an important decrease in blood pressure, whereas, if angiotensin II is not a factor in the etiology of a patient's hypertension, infusion of saralasin will not produce such a change.

The test is performed by titration of the blood pressure response to gradually increasing intravenous doses or by rapid administration of a single bolus. The former appears to be the safer method. A decrease in mean blood pressure of 5 to 10 mm Hg is considered clinically important and connotes a positive response.

The most serious problem associated with the saralasin test is a high incidence of false negative and false positive responses (about 15 to 20 per cent for both). Another problem is that saralasin acts as a partial agonist and may provoke an increase in blood pressure in patients with low plasma renin activity. Fortunately, the incidence of this potentially dangerous side effect is low, particularly if the dose is titrated. Finally, several medications may interfere with the renin-angiotensin system and confound interpretation of test results. To prevent this, one must withdraw drugs before the evaluation. In patients with severe hypertension, this should be done only in a hospital, and even then it may not be justified in terms of safety.

In our opinion, the use of saralasin may have some value in patients with strongly suspected renovascular hypertension in whom renal vein renin results are already known, and yet a question remains about selection for surgery. Thus, at the present time, we feel that the saralasin test, although of limited value, may in certain selective circumstances be useful in the diagnosis of renovascular hypertension.

If the screening tests are negative, antihypertensive medication should be initiated. If the patient is subsequently found to be refractory to drug therapy, it may be prudent to reconsider performing a renal arteriogram.

Assessment of Functional Significance of Renal Artery Stenosis

As noted earlier, the anatomic delineation of a renal arterial lesion by angiography in a hypertensive patient does not necessarily denote an etiologic relationship to the hypertension. It is incumbent upon the physician to demonstrate the functional significance of such a lesion. In the past, there was a flurry of enthusiasm for the use of peripheral PRA in assessing the physiologic significance of renal artery stenosis. Subsequent experience, however, has given rise to general dissatisfaction with the predictive value of peripheral

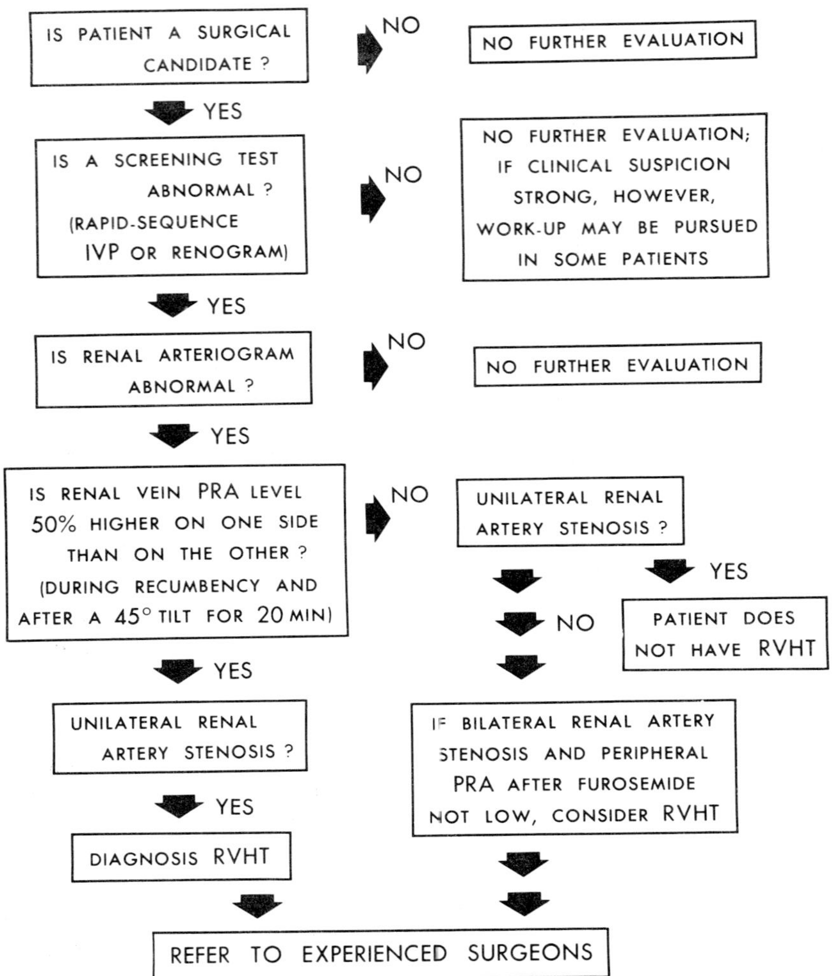

FIGURE 3–3. Evaluation of patients for renovascular hypertension (RVHT). IF RVHT is suspected clinically, the first consideration is whether the patient is a surgical candidate. If so, then the next step is the performance of a screening test, such as a rapid sequence IVP. Sometimes, if the clinical picture is strong, even if the IVP is negative, a renal arteriogram is done. In addition, some experts perform an arteriogram without a prior IVP. An abnormal arteriogram is followed by determination of bilateral renal vein renin levels. The importance of referral to experienced, competent surgeons cannot be overemphasized. (From Epstein, M, and Oster, J. *In* Halsted, JA, and Halsted, CH: The Laboratory in Clinical Medicine, 2nd ed. W. B. Saunders Co., Philadelphia, 1981.)

venous PRA, since normal values occur in patients with proven renovascular hypertension with a frequency exceeding 30 per cent. At present, renal vein PRA determinations are used widely for the identification of physiologically significant lesions. Unequivocal lateralization of increased renin concentration to the affected side indicates the possibility of cure or improvement of hypertension in more than 90 per cent of such patients. There has been some disagreement concerning the criterion for the ratio of renal vein PRA (affected side/contralateral side) to use in identifying *correctable* renovascular lesions in hypertensive patients. Nevertheless, most investigators cite a ratio of 1.5 or greater as indicative of lateralization to the affected kidney. A simplified flow diagram for the evaluation of renovascular hypertension is depicted in Figure 3–3.

Determining the Functional Significance of Renal Arterial Stenosis

It is not our intent to burden the clinician with the specifics of the protocols for the assessment of the functional significance of renal artery stenosis in general or for renal vein renin sampling in particular. Nevertheless, we believe that the clinician responsible for the primary care of patients with hypertension should have at least a general understanding of what is involved so that he can be in a position to evaluate rationally whether the consultant's recommendations for repair of renovascular hypertension are well founded and in the best interest of his patients.

Patients who undergo renal vein renin sampling should be carefully prepared for a standardized protocol. For example, assumption of upright posture may transiently augment renin release, with subsequent suppression of renin secretion during recumbency. Thus, to avoid obtaining confusing data, patients should remain recumbent overnight before the procedure. Similarly, medications that either decrease (e.g., beta-blockers) or increase (e.g., vasodilators) PRA should be avoided on the day of the procedure at a minimum, and if the patient's well-being is not compromised, preferably for one week before study.

Selective sampling from the renal veins requires an accurate determination of the site of the catheter tip. This is usually accomplished by injection of a small amount of radiopaque contrast medium. Blood should be obtained from all available renal veins. For example, to avoid dilution of the effluent from the ischemic segment by blood from the main renal vein, one must cannulate segmental veins in patients with segmental arterial lesions. Similarly, when sampling from the left kidney, one must advance the catheter so as to avoid sample dilution by blood emanating from the gonadal vein. Finally, sampling from the two kidneys and the inferior vena cava should be done in rapid succession so that the influence of factors that tend to cause fluctuations in PRA levels can be minimized.

When renal vein renin sampling is performed immediately after renal arteriography the first procedure may transiently either suppress or elevate PRA. Thus, if both procedures are to be done at one session, it is advisable to perform the renin sampling first. Alternatively, the patient can return for venous sampling if a lesion is demonstrated on arteriography.

Some investigators attempt to exaggerate the PRA differences between the normal and ischemic kidneys. This is accomplished either by tilting of the patient to a semi-upright position and intravenous administration of hydralazine, furosemide, or a converting enzyme inhibitor or by prior treatment with dietary sodium restriction and a diuretic.

Renal Parenchymal Disease

Chronic Renal Insufficiency. Hypertension complicates the course of the majority of patients whose chronic renal parenchymal disease has progressed to renal failure. Volume expansion, hyperreninemia, or both play important pathogenetic roles. Figure 3–4 summarizes in a schematic fashion the interrelationship of sodium, extracellular fluid volume, and the renin-angiotensin system in mediating the hypertension of patients with chronic renal insufficiency. According to this formulation, renal sodium retention causes expansion of ECF, increased cardiac output, and hypertension. The increase in blood pressure tends to augment sodium excretion, but this effect is insufficient to return the volume status to normal, and the renin-angiotensin-aldosterone axis is suppressed.

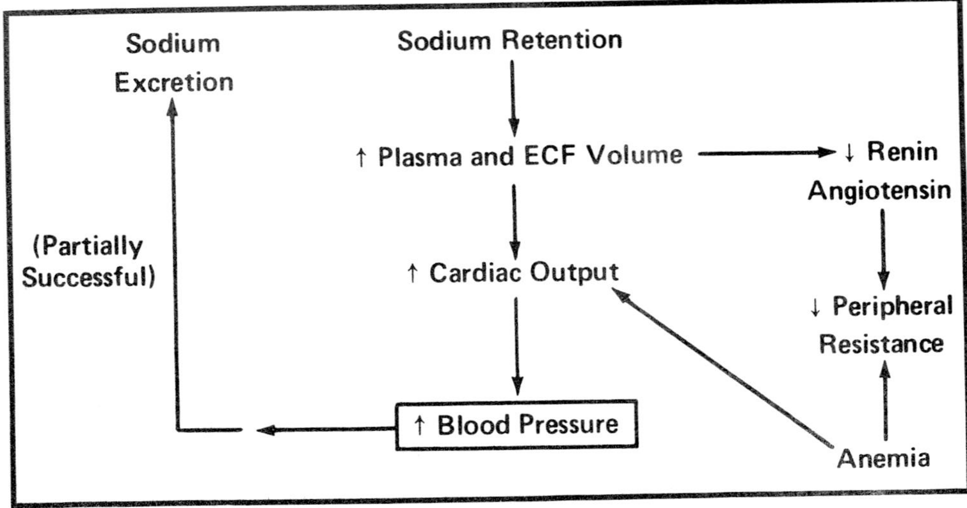

VOLUME—DEPENDENT OR CONTROLLABLE HYPERTENSION

FIGURE 3–4. The interrelationship of sodium, extracellular fluid volume (ECF), and the renin-angiotensin system in mediating the hypertension of patients with chronic renal insufficiency. According to this formulation, renal sodium retention causes expansion of ECF, increased cardiac output, and hypertension. The increase in blood pressure tends to augment sodium excretion, but this effect is insufficient to return the volume status to normal, and the renin-angiotensin-aldosterone axis is suppressed. (Reproduced with permission from Kaplan, NM: Clinical Hypertension, 3rd ed. The Williams & Wilkins Co., Baltimore, 1982.)

Patients with end-stage renal disease (ESRD) undergoing hemodialysis illustrate the dynamic interplay of these two factors. Since achievement of dry weight restores normotension in the great majority of patients (most of whom have normal PRA levels), the role of hypervolemia would appear obvious. On the other hand, plasma volume expansion may not adequately suppress PRA in some dialysis patients, so that the ratio of PRA to plasma volume in some is inappropriately high.

A small number of ESRD patients (10 to 15 per cent) have pure renin-dependent hypertension. These patients fail to achieve normal pressures despite restoration of dry weight; this group manifests marked persistent PRA elevation. In the past, nephrectomy was used to lower the blood pressure in these patients. Fortunately, this can now almost always be accomplished either with potent vasodilators such as minoxidil or by interference with the renin-angiotensin axis with drugs such as captopril.

Increased cardiac output, presumably as a response to anemia, is seen in many ESRD patients; along with deficiency of certain vasodepressors (e.g., prostaglandins) from the renal medulla, it may add to the hypertension.

In summary, the hypertension in ESRD patients is multifactorial and may relate to hypervolemia, increased cardiac output, enhanced vascular sensitivity to angiotensin (secondary to sodium retention), and failure of diseased ischemic kidneys to suppress renin secretion totally.

Acute Glomerulonephritis. Up to 75 per cent of patients with acute poststreptococcal glomerulonephritis manifest edema and hypertension. Volume overload and increased cardiac output are major factors elevating the blood pressure. Since the PRA of such patients is not totally suppressed, one could argue that a "normal" value in the face of volume expansion reflects an inappropriately "elevated" value.

Obstructive Uropathy. Bilateral ureteral obstruction is a well-known but quite uncommon cause of hypertension. Its pathogenesis is similar to that of other forms of renal insufficiency: volume overload with inappropriately high levels of renin. Unilateral hydronephrosis also may produce a curable form of hypertension quite similar in pathogenesis to renovascular hypertension. The total body sodium is normal in these patients, suggesting that volume expansion does not play a major role.

Juxtaglomerular Cell Tumors and Other Renin-producing Tumors. Juxtaglomerular cell tumors (hemangiopericytomas) and Wilms' tumors are rare causes of renal hypertension. Both neoplasms may secrete large amounts of renin. The PRA levels are extraordinarily high in the venous drainage of the tumor-laden kidney. Cure may be effected by nephrectomy or selective excision of the tumor.

Unilateral Renal Disease. Whether unilateral renal parenchymal disease is an important cause of hypertension is unsettled. Nephrectomy restores normotension in only 26 per cent of hypertensive patients with unilaterally small kidneys. Furthermore, many of these patients might have had unilaterally small kidneys secondary to renal artery stenosis. The majority of patients reported with nonvascular unilateral disease have had either pyelonephritis or hydronephrosis. Most of those with pyelonephritis failed to demonstrate elevated PRA levels, lateralizing renal vein renin ratios, or contralateral renal renin suppression. Thus, the hypertension may have been essential, and the unilateral parenchymal disease might have been coincidental. Other explanations include unrecognized bilateral renal disease or the release by the kidney of an as yet unidentified pressor substance.

Mineralocorticoid-induced Hypertension

Some of the more frequently encountered forms of mineralocorticoid-related hypertension are listed in Table 3–1. Primary aldosteronism, or "low-renin hyperaldosteronism," is the most important of these; other types of mineralocorticoid excess include Cushing's syndrome, adrenogenital syndrome, and licorice abuse. Primary aldosteronism is characterized by the excessive production of aldosterone (typically by an adrenal adenoma), resulting in renal sodium retention, kaliuresis, hypokalemia, and hypochloremic metabolic alkalosis. The hyperaldosteronism is not suppressible by saline administration. As intravascular volume increases, blood pressure rises (Fig. 3–5). As a result of volume expansion, PRA tends to be suppressed and to respond sluggishly to stimulatory maneuvers (i.e., dietary sodium restriction, furosemide administration). The hypertension associated with primary aldosteronism usually responds well to either the administration of the mineralocorticoid antagonist spironolactone or surgical removal of the adenoma.

Primary aldosteronism is not a common cause of hypertension. Conn originally postulated that normokalemic cases might account for as many as 20 per cent of patients with apparent essential hypertension, but it quickly became apparent that this was a gross overestimate of the frequency. For example, Berglund and his associates in Sweden, using potassium measurements for screening, found only one case among 689 hypertensive men.

Symptoms. It should be emphasized that some patients have no relevant symptoms, and present for a routine evaluation or an incidental complaint with

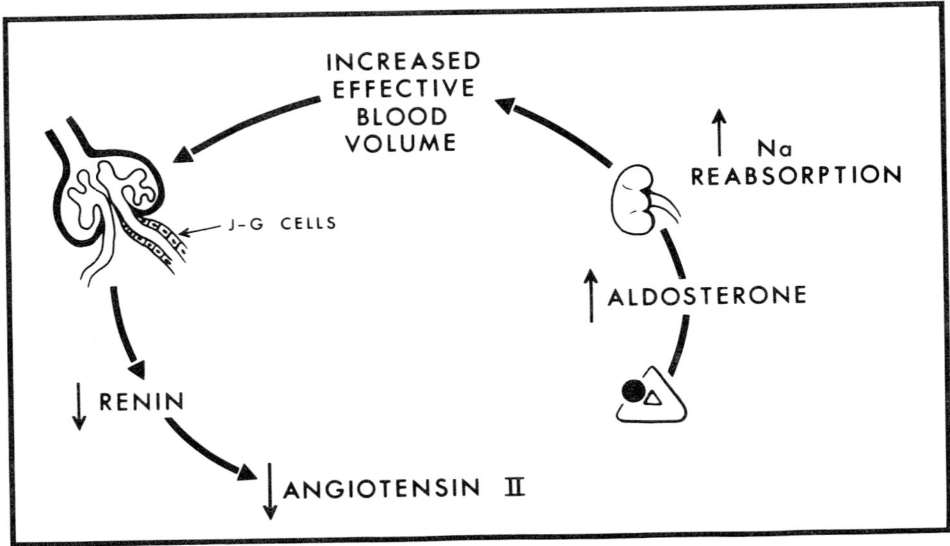

FIGURE 3–5. Alterations in the renin-angiotensin-aldosterone system in primary aldosteronism. The initiating event is an excessive secretion of aldosterone due to a defect in the adrenal cortex *(lower right corner)*. As a result of chronic excessive secretion of aldosterone, a mild expansion of ECF volume ensues with elevation of blood pressure. As a consequence of volume expansion, plasma renin activity and angiotensin II are suppressed markedly.

hypertension. Conversely, patients may present with symptoms of hypokalemia, such as muscle weakness, polyuria, nocturia, and polydipsia, and less commonly with paresthesias or actual muscle paralysis. Headache is also common.

Figure 3–6 depicts the major metabolic features of excessive aldosterone production that ultimately account for the clinical presentation of primary aldosteronism. Renal potassium wasting is the classic manifestation of aldosterone excess. Not surprisingly, this feature is often exaggerated by administration of thiazide-type diuretics and ameliorated by the administration of the mineralocorticoid antagonist spironolactone. The other important phenomenon highlighted by the figure is that maneuvers that either augment or diminish the delivery of sodium to the distal nephron will simultaneously aggravate or diminish renal potassium wasting. As an example, dietary sodium restriction, which results in a diminution of distal sodium delivery, minimizes urinary potassium losses. Conversely, a high sodium intake exaggerates renal potassium wasting by increasing the delivery of sodium to sites in the distal nephron that are aldosterone responsive.

Some of the other clinical laboratory findings of mineralocorticoid excess depend in part on both the severity and the duration of potassium depletion. For example, the degree of hypochloremic metabolic alkalosis (which is caused primarily by increased renal ammonium excretion) appears to correlate with the severity of hypokalemia. Similarly, marked potassium depletion may impair the ability of the kidney to conserve water, and this results in mild polyuria and polydipsia. Concomitant water loss and sodium retention probably account for the frequent finding of mild hypernatremia.

Although it was originally stated that the hypertension of primary aldosteronism is comparatively mild, this concept is no longer valid. Most experts now believe that the blood pressure may be markedly elevated in primary hyperaldosteronism. Indeed, Ferriss and his associates from Glasgow have

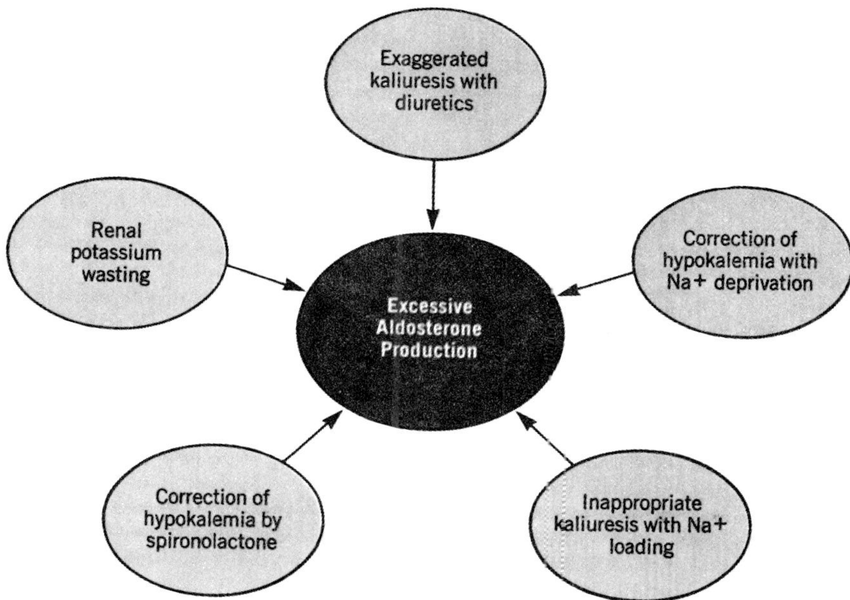

FIGURE 3–6. Important features of renal potassium wasting associated with mineralocorticoid excess. Not surprisingly, potassium depletion is exaggerated by the use of non–potassium-sparing diuretics or increased sodium intake, and is minimized by administration of the mineralocorticoid antagonist spironolactone or dietary sodium restriction. (Reproduced with permission from G. D. Searle & Co.: Clinician [Hypertension], 1973.)

reported that the mean blood pressure of their patients was 205/123 mm Hg ± 28/13 (SD).

Classification of Primary Aldosteronism. The first described patient with primary aldosteronism was found to have an adrenocortical adenoma, but this syndrome may be attributable to a number of other abnormalities, some of them quite rare. A classification of primary aldosteronism is shown in Table 3–5.

Unilateral, or rarely bilateral, adrenal adenoma is believed to be by far the most common cause of primary aldosteronism, usually constituting about 85 to 90 per cent of published series. Some of the more recently reported studies, however, have found an increased incidence (as high as 30 per cent or more) of other etiologies. Patients with bilateral adrenal cortical hyperplasia (so-called idiopathic hyperaldosteronism) make up most of these; unfortunately, surgery does not cure patients with this form of the syndrome. Rarely, patients with aldosterone excess are found to have glucocorticoid-responsive hyperaldoster-

TABLE 3–5.   TYPES OF PRIMARY HYPERALDOSTERONISM

MOST COMMON

1. Aldosterone-producing adrenocortical adenoma (Conn's syndrome)
2. Idiopathic hyperaldosteronism (nodular hyperplasia of zona glomerulosa)

RARE

3. Glucocorticoid-responsive hyperaldosteronism
4. Aldosterone-producing adrenocortical carcinoma
5. Aldosterone-producing ovarian carcinoma

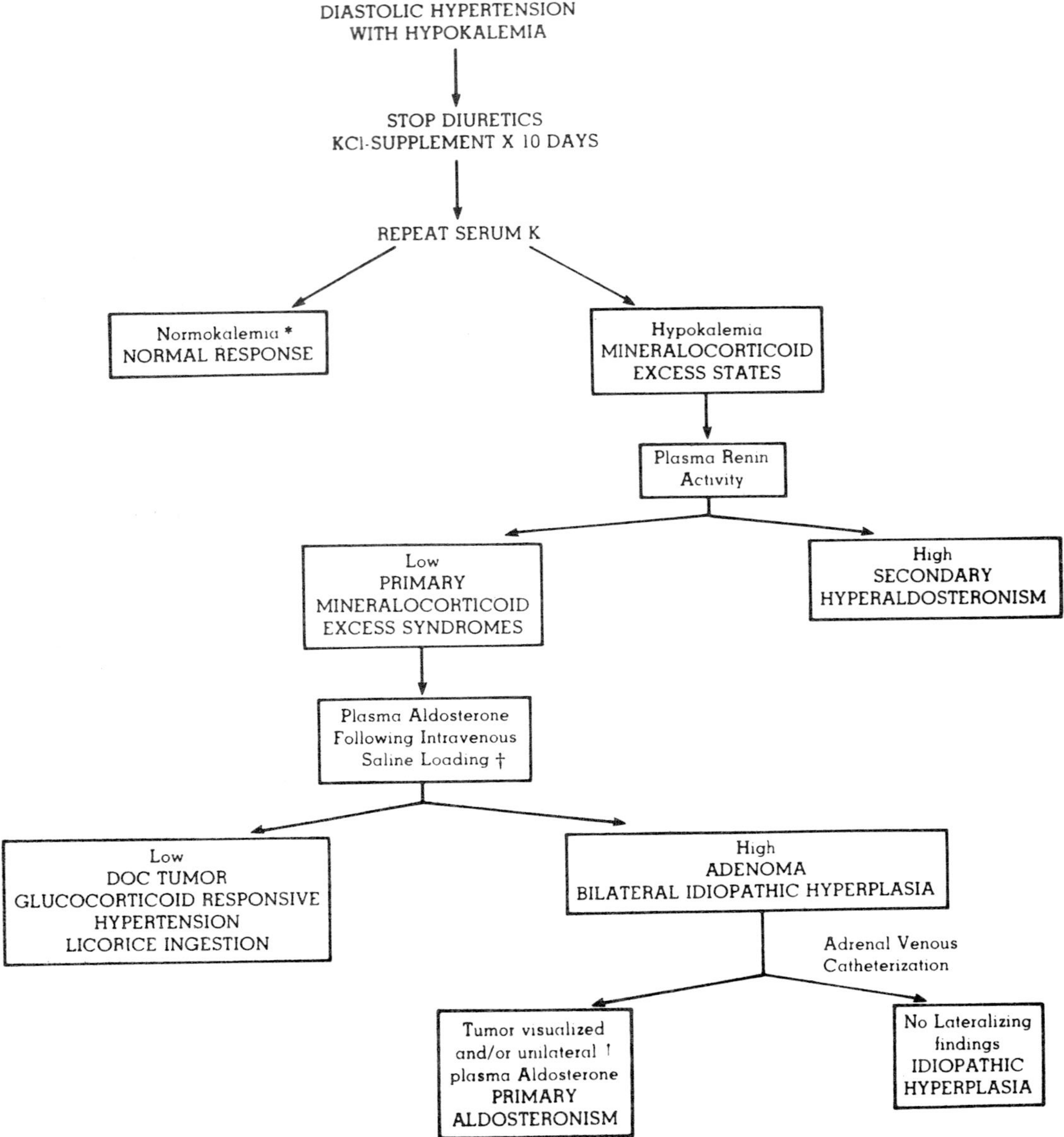

FIGURE 3–7. Algorithm for the evaluation of patients with suspected primary aldosteronism. As can be seen, the patient is categorized initially with respect to his serum potassium level. If hypokalemia persists despite discontinuation of diuretics, plasma renin activity is determined to assess whether the patient has primary or secondary hyperaldosteronism. High PRA levels indicate secondary hyperaldosteronism, whereas suppressed levels suggest one of several primary mineralocorticoid excess syndromes. (Reproduced with permission from Isselbacher, KJ, et al.: Harrison's Principles of Internal Medicine, 9th ed. McGraw-Hill Book Co., New York, 1979.)

onism. Patients with this syndrome usually present with the typical features of hypertension, hypokalemia, aldosterone excess, and low PRA. The condition may be familial, apparently with an autosomal dominant transmission. Glucocorticoids such as dexamethasone produce a sustained reversal of all the abnormalities, usually within two weeks. In glucocorticoid-suppressible hyperaldosteronism, the postural response of plasma aldosterone is similar to that found in patients with adenomas. Spironolactone and adrenalectomy usually do not significantly improve the hypertension.

Other rare entities include indeterminant hyperaldosteronism and hyper-aldosteronism associated with adrenal cortical carcinoma or ovarian neoplasms.

The Evaluation for Primary Aldosteronism. Figures 3–7, 3–8, and 3–9 illustrate the diagnostic considerations that relate to work-up of primary aldosteronism. Suspicion that mineralocorticoid excess may be responsible for the elevated blood pressure of a patient is frequently aroused by the presence of unprovoked hypokalemia. As noted earlier, the effects of aldosterone excess result in an initial period of expansion of extracellular fluid volume with a persistent urinary wastage of potassium. As a consequence, hypokalemia develops. Although the majority (60 to 90 per cent) of patients with primary aldosteronism manifest hypokalemia, many, particularly those who are taking potassium-sparing diuretics or ingesting low sodium–high potassium diets, may have normal potassium levels. In the study of Bravo et al. (1983), 28 per cent of patients ingesting a regular sodium diet were normokalemic, and approximately half of these remained so despite three days of salt loading.

In approaching the patient with hypertension and hypokalemia, the clinician may be presented with a dilemma if the serum potassium level was not measured before initiation of chronic diuretic therapy. After discontinuation of thiazides, the patient should be instructed to ingest a normal amount of sodium and avoid potassium supplementation other than in the diet. At the end of a 7-to-10–day period, a 24-hour urine should be collected for determination of sodium and potassium content, and a repeat serum potassium determined. If the patient's hypokalemia has lessened (or been corrected), and the urine contains at least 100 mEq of sodium and less than 30 mEq of potassium, it is unlikely that aldosteronism is present (Figs. 3–7 and 3–8). Rather, one presumes that the hypokalemia was thiazide induced and may require several more days for spontaneous correction. If, however, the urinary potassium exceeds 30

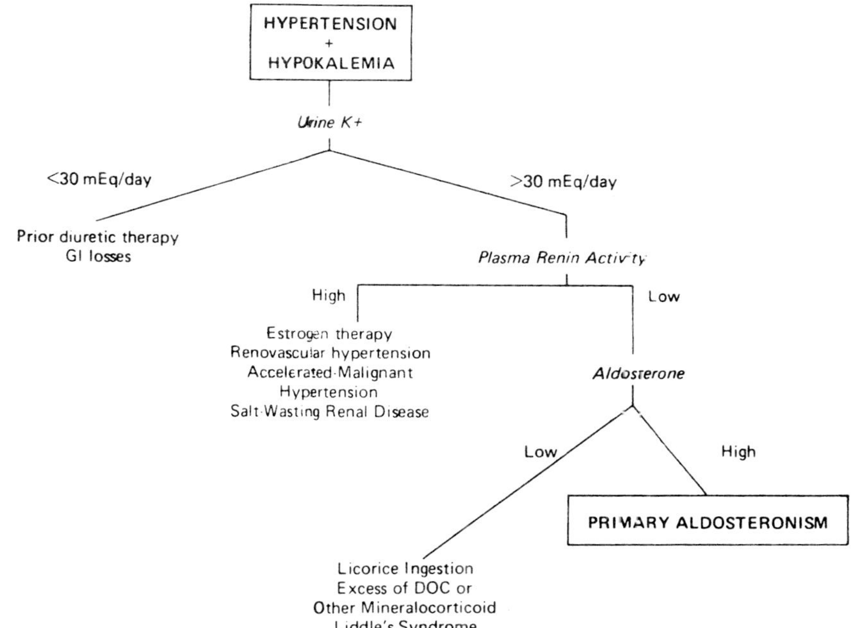

FIGURE 3–8. Flow diagram for diagnostic work-up of hypertensive patients with hypokalemia. (Reproduced with permission from Kaplan, NM: Clinical Hypertension, 3rd ed. The Williams & Wilkins Co., Baltimore, 1982.)

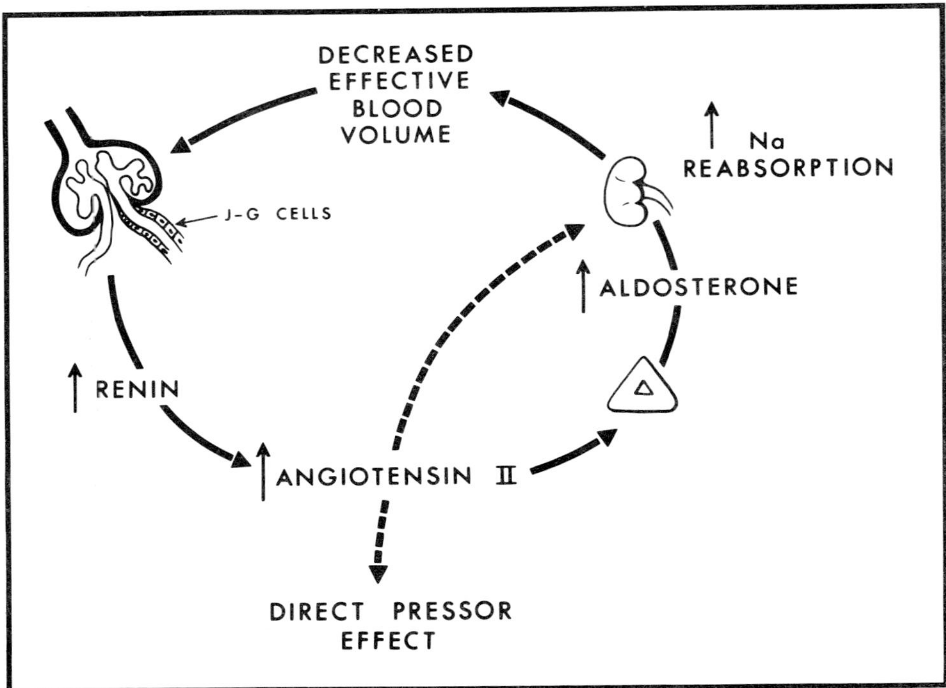

FIGURE 3–9. The renin-angiotensin-aldosterone system in secondary hyperaldosteronism. The initiating event is thought to be a decrease in *effective* circulating blood volume. As a result, several mechanisms are brought into play favoring facilitation of renin release. Chronic stimulation of the renin-angiotensin axis leads to an excessive production of aldosterone. Measurement of PRA constitutes one of the most important determinations in distinguishing between *primary* and *secondary* hyperaldosteronism. (See also Fig. 3–5.)

mEq/day and the patient is still hypokalemic, additional diagnostic evaluation is necessary, since the patient probably has aldosteronism or another disease causing renal potassium wastage (Figs. 3–7 and 3–8). If hypertension is severe (diastolic pressure 110 to 115 mm Hg or greater), or if cardiac failure is present, the potential risk does not warrant withdrawal of diuretic therapy unless another (nondiuretic) medication has been started.

The attempt to establish the diagnosis of primary aldosteronism is predicated on the realization that hypersecretion of aldosterone associated with hypertension may be due either to autonomous hyperfunction of the adrenal cortex (primary aldosteronism) or to excessive stimulation of the renin-angiotensin axis (secondary aldosteronism) (Fig. 3–9). Determination of PRA is helpful in separating the hypertension associated with hyperaldosteronism into these two types. Patients with primary aldosteronism typically manifest suppressed PRA levels (Fig. 3–5), which respond poorly to stimulatory maneuvers, including upright posture, dietary sodium deprivation, or intravenous administration of diazoxide or furosemide. Furthermore, PRA measurements may be helpful in differentiating between adenomatous and nonadenomatous forms of primary aldosteronism.

Although the demonstration of low PRA levels is a useful screening test, it should be emphasized that such a finding *alone* does not establish the diagnosis of primary aldosteronism, since PRA is also suppressed in 25 per cent of essential hypertensives (see p. 40). In addition, Bravo et al. (1983) observed that 28 per cent of their patients had a normal or elevated PRA while ingesting a normal sodium intake. Furthermore, the authors had previously shown that diuretic-treated patients with adrenal cortical adenomas have PRA levels that are indistinguishable from those of patients with essential hypertension.

Classically, the autonomy of aldosterone excess in primary aldosteronism has been established by the demonstration of *both suppressed PRA* (despite the stimulation of sodium depletion) *and inappropriately elevated aldosterone levels* (relative to the expected values in a sodium-replete state). The responsiveness of plasma aldosterone may be assessed by the infusion of saline. Alternative methods for assessing the nonsuppressibility of aldosterone secretion include oral sodium loading (200 mEq/day for three days) or 10 mg deoxycorticosterone acetate (DOCA) intramuscularly every 12 hours for three days while the patient ingests a regular diet. Hypokalemia should be corrected before volume expansion because potassium depletion may result in some reduction of plasma aldosterone, even in a patient with an adenoma.

Because of high rates of both false-positive and false-negative results, Bravo et al. consider that measurements of serum potassium and PRA are inadequate screening tests. In their hands, the best sensitivity (95 per cent) and specificity (93 per cent) in identifying patients with primary aldosteronism was conferred by the demonstration of excessive aldosterone production after three days of salt loading. Hypokalemia, suppressed PRA, or both were considered corroborative but not necessary findings. In an outpatient, the physician may add 10 to 12 g of salt per day to the patient's diet and measure 24-hour excretion of sodium, potassium, and aldosterone after five to seven days. The urine sodium excretion should be at least 250 mEq/day as evidence of an adequate sodium intake.

Once the provisional diagnosis of a probable adrenocortical adenoma is made, an attempt should be made to localize the lesion anatomically. In the series of Bravo et al., the measurement of adrenal venous plasma aldosterone proved to be 100 per cent accurate as a localizing procedure. The authors recommend that a computerized axial tomographic (CAT) scan be done first and, if positive, be considered diagnostic. Adrenal venous sampling should be carried out if the results of the scan are inconclusive.

Methods for Differentiating Between the Adenomatous and Idiopathic Forms. Differentiation between the two principal forms of primary aldosterone excess, aldosterone-producing adenoma and idiopathic hyperaldosteronism (i.e., hyperplastic form), is of considerable clinical importance. Not only is the pathogenesis distinct, but treatment is often different. In particular, adrenal surgery is usually indicated for patients in the former group, whereas patients with idiopathic hyperaldosteronism are treated medically since surgery is not corrective. Various methods of distinguishing the two forms have been advocated, including the statistical technique of quadric analysis. For a more detailed consideration of this complicated subject, the reader is referred to the extensive review by Ferriss et al. (1970).

Biochemical abnormalities are often greater in patients with adenoma as opposed to those in patients with hyperplasia. Thus, mean plasma (and urinary) levels for aldosterone, sodium and bicarbonate tend to be significantly higher and those of potassium and PRA significantly lower in the adenoma group. Such findings, however, are not universal. Similarly, an anomalous postural decrease in plasma aldosterone has also been reported in the majority of patients with a unilateral adenoma, but this test is of limited diagnostic value in the individual patient.

In the study of Bravo et al. (1983), the best indicators of the presence of an adenoma (versus hyperplasia) were severe persistent hypokalemia, a postural decrease in plasma aldosterone, and an increased plasma level of 18-hydroxycorticosterone. A definitive diagnosis can often be made by preoperative, bilateral cannulation of the adrenal veins; patients with adenoma demonstrate either unilateral increments in plasma aldosterone concentration, tumor visualization on the involved side, or both features.

Low-Renin "Essential" Hypertension

It has been estimated that 20 to 25 per cent of patients with apparent essential hypertension manifest suppression of the renin-angiotensin system. The mechanism underlying this unresponsiveness to stimuli that normally increase renin remains undefined. Although some observers have speculated that excessive secretion of an as yet unidentified mineralocorticoid may be responsible for both the suppression of renin and the hypertension, others believe that it is more likely that the majority of such cases reflect long-term renal adaptations to hypertension. Although early work suggested that aldosterone antagonists constituted specific treatment for such patients, subsequent studies have demonstrated that other diuretics that are not specific mineralocorticoid antagonists are equally effective. These observations underscore the fact that blood pressure reduction depends primarily on volume reduction rather than on specific antagonism of excessive mineralocorticoid effect.

The past several years have witnessed increasing interest in the pathophysiologic and therapeutic implications of the renin status of patients with essential hypertension. Laragh and his associates have suggested that the probability of patients' developing major vascular complications of essential hypertension is directly related to their renin status. It was proposed that low renin levels protect against vascular complications of hypertension. Implicit in such a thesis is the assumption that antihypertensive drugs that raise renin levels may prove to be harmful and that choice of the optimal agent for the treatment of a hypertensive requires knowledge of the renin status of the patient. In contrast to these early observations, many subsequent studies have shown that patients with low renin values are just as susceptible to vascular complications as those with normal levels. In addition, the suggestion that prior knowledge of the renin status of patients with essential hypertension facilitates subsequent drug therapy has come under criticism and is not widely accepted.

As a result of this continuing controversy, many practitioners are having difficulty in deciding whether they should perform renin assays on their hypertensive patients in order to determine prognosis and therapeutic approach. Despite the provocative hypotheses regarding the renin status of hypertensive patients, we believe that it is inappropriate to extrapolate this formulation to all hypertensive patients. The potential advantage of choosing antihypertensive agents on the basis of renin status remains problematic, and there are clear-cut difficulties in the practical application of this hypothesis. Thus, the general adoption by practicing clinicians of a policy of determining the renin status of hypertensive patients could involve additional costs, subject millions of hypertensive patients to additional risks from unnecessary procedures, and delay treatment with safe and effective drugs.

Hypertension Associated with Hormonal Contraceptives

Prospective controlled studies have shown that estrogen-progestogen oral contraceptives (containing 50 μg or more of estrogen) cause a distinct, albeit small, increase in systolic pressure in virtually all women. In some individuals marked elevation of pressure can occur, and occasional patients have been seen in the malignant phase. Almost invariably the pressure falls when the oral contraceptive is withdrawn.

The mechanism whereby the "pill" induces a rise in blood pressure is imperfectly understood. It is well known that estrogens increase hepatic synthesis of renin substrate (Fig. 3–2), and many authors have invoked aberrations of the renin-angiotensin system as the mechanism whereby the pill induces hypertension. Recent studies have indicated that PRA is elevated in most subjects taking the pill, regardless of their blood pressure. It is thus apparent that the true role of the renin-angiotensin system in mediating hypertension of the pill is uncertain, and much additional work is necessary to elucidate the relationship further.

Although the mechanism(s) whereby the pill is associated with hypertension remains undefined, the effects of the pill cannot be ignored. First, the current consensus is that oral contraceptives should not be prescribed to patients with a history of hypertension. Furthermore, it is incumbent upon the physician who places his patient on an estrogen preparation or oral contraceptive to monitor the blood pressure frequently and to discontinue these preparations immediately should the patient become hypertensive. In addition, the alterations in PRA and aldosterone induced by the pill may simulate curable forms of hypertension such as renovascular hypertension. Thus, any work-up for renovascular hypertension or primary aldosteronism should be performed after discontinuation of all estrogen-progestogen medications for at least one month.

Pheochromocytoma

Although pheochromocytoma constitutes a very infrequent cause of hypertension, it merits consideration and discussion because its pathophysiology is perhaps the best understood of all the hypertensive diseases and because its therapy, when successful, is the surest. Although the precise incidence of pheochromocytoma is unknown, as many as 0.1 per cent of the population with diastolic hypertension might have this tumor. If one assumes an incidence of 0.1 per cent in Americans with sustained diastolic hypertension, there may be 50,000 persons or more harboring the tumor in the United States.

Pheochromocytomas are chromaffin cell tumors that can arise wherever these cells are found, i.e., mainly in the adrenal medulla but also within the sympathetic ganglia and paraganglia that lie along the sympathetic chain. It has been estimated that as many as 80 to 90 per cent of pheochromocytomas are found in one or both adrenal glands. The features of catecholamine excess secondary to pheochromocytomas are frequently dramatic, mandating the attention of the clinician. In fact, pheochromocytoma is perhaps the most fascinating of all tumors. Its clinical expressions, often dramatic and explosive, are so variable that it has rightly earned the title of the "great mimic." A majority of patients with pheochromocytoma have either headache, sweating, or palpitations, and many have all three in association with paroxysms.

Although paroxysms are often thought to represent the classic feature of pheochromocytoma, it should be noted that truly paroxysmal hypertension,

**TABLE 3–6. FREQUENCY OF COMMON SYMPTOMS AND SIGNS OF
PHEOCHROMOCYTOMA**

Hypertension—probably over 98%
  Intermittent only—2 to 50%
  Sustained—50 to 60%
  Paroxysms superimposed—about 50%
Headache—80 to 85%
Sweating—65 to 70%
Palpitations—60 to 65%
Nervousness—35 to 40%
Nausea and vomiting—35 to 60%
Weight loss—40 to 70%
Funduscopic changes—50 to 70%

Modified from Kaplan, NM: Clinical Hypertension, 3rd ed. The Williams & Wilkins Co., Baltimore, 1982.

with intervening normotension, is relatively unusual; more than half of patients with pheochromocytoma have *sustained* hypertension. The most common symptoms and signs are summarized in Table 3–6. Symptoms of pheochromocytoma are due either to pharmacologic effects of excessive concentrations of circulating catecholamines or to complications of hypertension induced by these pressor amines. The three most commonly experienced symptoms in patients with either paroxysmal or persistent hypertension are headache, excessive sweating, and palpitations.

Headaches are almost always paroxysmal in character, are frequently throbbing and bilateral, and are usually very severe during a paroxysm of hypertension.

About two-thirds of patients have excessive perspiration (sometimes "drenching" in nature) that is generalized, but more so in the upper body and not confined to one area. The most profuse sweating appears during paroxysmal attacks of hypertension.

Palpitations, the third most common symptom, are usually accompanied by tachycardia, although sometimes reflex bradycardia may be elicited by the increased blood pressure. Patients frequently complain of "pounding" in the chest, sometimes severe enough to be described as "like a sledge hammer" or as if the heart were going to burst through the ribs.

When features suggestive of pheochromocytoma are present, the diagnosis can be established with relative ease as compared with other forms of secondary hypertension. The sine qua non for preoperative diagnosis of pheochromocytoma is demonstration of elevated catecholamines, their metabolites, or both, in urine or demonstration of elevated plasma catecholamines. Reliability of the assay is mandatory. Exploratory surgery to locate a catecholamine-secreting tumor without chemical or radiologic evidence of a tumor is indefensible.

When the physician decides to measure the excretion of catecholamines and their metabolites, the conditions of sampling must be borne in mind. It is worth emphasizing that the patient should be instructed to avoid severe stress, which may result in significantly elevated levels of the substances assayed.

Conditions other than pheochromocytoma and medication use that may be accompanied by significantly increased or decreased excretion of catecholamines and their metabolites are indicated in Table 3–7. Tests are readily available for each of the three urinary products of catecholamine metabolism, i.e., metanephrine + normetanephrine, free catecholamines, and vanillylmandelic acid (VMA). The first-mentioned constitutes the most expeditious and

TABLE 3–7. INTERFERING FACTORS IN BIOCHEMICAL DETERMINATIONS FOR DIAGNOSIS OF PHEOCHROMOCYTOMA

Free Catecholamines (norepinephrine and epinephrine)	Metanephrines and Normetanephrines	VMA
A. ANALYTIC FACTORS *Increase* Tetracycline Quinidine Quinine Chloral hydrate (non-specific fluorescence) *Decrease* None described B. PHARMACOLOGIC FACTORS *Increase* Methyldopa (Aldomet) Levodopa (Larodopa, Dopar) Isoproterenol Theophylline Prochlorperazine (Compazine) Strenuous exercise Hypoglycemia *Decrease* Clonidine (Catapres)	A. ANALYTIC FACTORS *Increase* Chlorpromazine *Decrease* X-ray contrast media containing methylglucamine (e.g., Renografin, Renovist, Hypaque, Conray) B. PHARMACOLOGIC FACTORS *Increase* MAO inhibitors Methyldopa (variable) *Decrease* None described	A. ANALYTIC FACTORS *Increase* Nalidixic acid (NegGram) *Decrease* Clofibrate (Atromid) B. PHARMACOLOGIC FACTORS *Increase* (all slight) Levodopa Lithium Nitroglycerin *Decrease* MAO inhibitors Methyldopa

Modified from Kaplan, NM: Clinical Hypertension, 3rd ed. The Williams & Wilkins Co., Baltimore, 1982.

simplest of the three tests, and is relatively free from interference by most medications and food ingredients. Furthermore, since the excretion of metanephrines is relatively constant (in contrast to the diurnal variation of free catecholamine excretion), and in view of the frequent problems in collecting *accurate* 24-hour urine specimens, the metanephrine assay lends itself to the collection of a single voided specimen with the results expressed per milligram of creatinine. Although the assay for total catecholamines is more difficult to perform, some workers suggest that it is practical to measure both total catecholamines and metanephrine in the initial screening procedure. This increases the sensitivity from 70 to 80 per cent to over 90 per cent.

Many investigators believe that it may not be necessary to fractionate total catecholamines into epinephrine and norepinephrine, although fractionation has been utilized to help localize the tumor (the CAT scan has currently superseded this approach). On the other hand, although uncommon, the level of either epinephrine or norepinephrine can be increased, whereas their sum may be within the normal range.

When an abnormal value is obtained by the metanephrine or VMA assay, measurement of free catecholamines (epinephrine and norepinephrine) should be carried out to confirm the abnormality. Furthermore, this procedure is helpful in the localization of the pheochromocytoma, since the documentation of excessive production of epinephrine alone suggests that the tumor probably resides in the adrenal glands.

Single- and double-isotope derivative methods for plasma catecholamine determinations have been developed and have recently become available in a number of clinical laboratories. Some of these assays provide reliable and sensitive data, but there are problems with the interpretation of the results that do not at present commend the use of plasma catecholamine assays for the diagnosis of pheochromocytoma. For example, plasma levels may fluctuate markedly, and repeated samplings are often required. In addition, it is clear that patients with essential hypertension and high renin levels may have markedly elevated plasma norepinephrine levels that tend to overlap those observed in patients with pheochromocytoma. Although plasma catecholamine determinations are not generally recommended for the diagnosis of pheochromocytoma, they may prove to be useful in the preoperative localization of extra-adrenal tumors. Multiple blood samples drawn from various levels of the inferior vena cava can be used to localize the tumor(s) after the diagnosis of pheochromocytoma has been established by urinary assays.

In 90 to 95 per cent of patients the diagnosis of pheochromocytoma can be established with ease when typical signs and symptoms (e.g., hypertension, sweating, palpitation, and headaches) are associated with unequivocal biochemical evidence of excessive catecholamine production. On the other hand, excluding the diagnosis in the 5 to 10 per cent of patients with essential hypertension who have suggestive symptoms and borderline increases in plasma catecholamines, urinary catecholamine metabolites, or both remains a common problem. Since a physiologic increase in catecholamines depends on activation of the sympathetic nervous system, whereas release from a tumor is presumed to be autonomous, specific inhibition of neurogenically mediated catecholamine release would differentiate sympathetic hyperactivity from pheochromocytoma.

It should be emphasized that in view of the widespread availability of accurate urinary assays for diagnosing pheochromocytoma, the role for pharmacologic tests, whether provocative (such as those involving administration of histamine, tyramine, or glucagon) or blocking (administration of phentolamine [Regitine]) tests, is limited. Some of these tests involve significant risks, including hypertensive crisis, and are fraught with an unacceptable level of false positive and false negative results. On the other hand, a preliminary report suggests that a newly described pharmacologic test, the clonidine suppression test, may be both accurate and safe. It has been proposed that the administration of a single oral dose of clonidine is a useful adjunctive to rule out pheochromocytoma in hypertensive patients with suggestive symptoms and borderline catecholamine values. In normal individuals and those with essential hypertension, clonidine suppresses plasma norepinephrine levels, possibly by stimulating central alpha-2 adrenergic receptors. Despite the apparent attractiveness of this test, its value remains to be determined.

A flow diagram for the evaluation of a patient for pheochromocytoma is shown in Figure 3–10. It should be noted that the clinical picture may be suggested not only by characteristic clinical manifestations but sometimes by hypertension that is particularly resistant to therapy.

Once the diagnosis of pheochromocytoma is confirmed by chemical analysis, it is important for the surgeon to know the precise location and extent of the tumor in order to effect its safe and expeditious removal. Selective arteriography is commonly used, since it can accurately demonstrate the blood supply and extent of most pheochromocytomas, but it is an invasive procedure with serious potential complications, including, rarely, hypertensive crisis. Adrenal vein and inferior vena cava blood sampling for catecholamines can help localize tumors in selected patients, but these are also invasive procedures

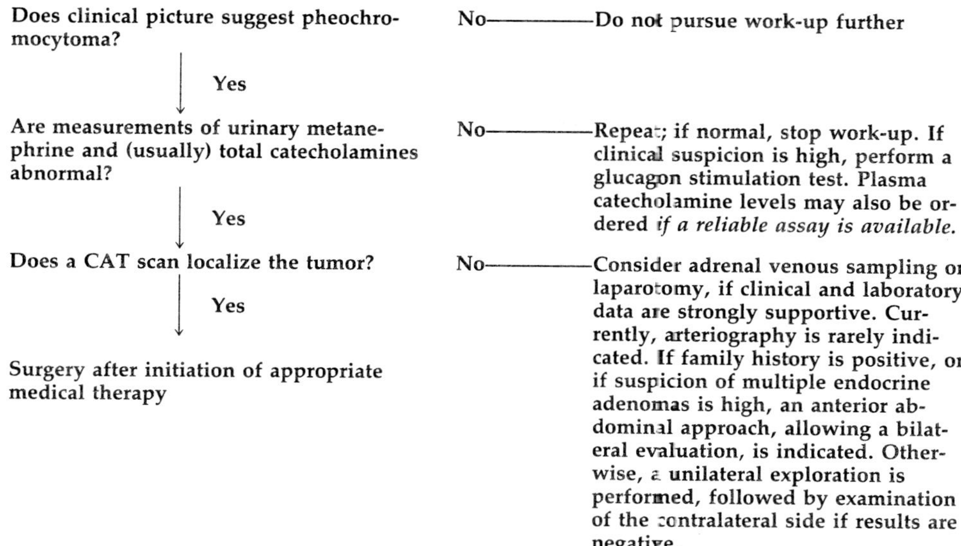

FIGURE 3–10. Algorithm for the evaluation of pheochromocytoma. If pheochromocytoma is suspected clinically, the appropriate urinary hormonal determinations should be performed, sometimes supplemented by specific catecholamine assays. Plasma assay and the clonidine suppression test may have a place in the difficult case. Finally, anatomic assessment with the CAT scan or other maneuvers for tumor localization is done if biochemical evaluation is positive or the clinical picture is highly suggestive of pheochromocytoma.

and of little help in estimating the size and extent of disease. Several recent reports indicate that pheochromocytomas can be localized effectively by CAT scanning. This technique has for the most part supplanted arteriography in the preoperative localization of pheochromocytoma.

Even though the symptoms of pheochromocytoma can be controlled medically (see Chapter 14), almost all observers feel that surgery is indicated because a significant number of the tumors may be malignant (as many as 10 per cent). Furthermore, the majority of patients with pheochromocytoma are cured by surgery, thereby obviating the necessity for lifelong medical therapy.

REFERENCES

Tucker, RM, and Labarthe, DM: Frequency of surgical treatment for hypertension in adults at the Mayo clinic from 1973 through 1975. Mayo Clin Proc 52:549–555, 1977.

Davis, BA, Crook, JE, Vestal, RE, and Oates, JA: Prevalence of renovascular hypertension in patients with grade III or IV hypertensive retinopathy. N Engl J Med 301:1273–1276, 1979.

Brown, JJ, Davies, DL, Morton, JJ, Robertson, JIS, Cuesta, V, Lever, AF, Padfield, PL, Trust, P, Bianchi, G, and Schalekamp, MAD: Mechanism of renal hypertension. Lancet I:1219–1221, 1976.

Perloff, D, and Schambelan, M: Renovascular hypertension. Clin Endocrinol Metab 10:513–535, 1981.

Vaughan, ED, Jr: Renal artery stenosis. In Hypertension. Contemporary Issues in Nephrology, vol. 8. Churchill Livingstone, New York, 1981, pp. 247–269.

Diagnosis of Renovascular Hypertension

Grim, CE, Luft, FC, Weinberger, MH, and Grim, CM: Sensitivity and specificity of screening tests for renal vascular hypertension. Ann Intern Med 91:617–622, 1979.

Maxwell, MH, Marks, LS, Lupu, AN, Cahill, PJ, Franklin, SS, and Kaufman, JJ: Predictive value of renin determinations in renal artery stenosis. JAMA 238:2617–2620, 1977.

Vaughan, ED, Jr, Buhler, FR, and Laragh, JH: Renovascular hypertension: renin measurements to indicate hypersecretion and contralateral suppression, estimate renal plasma flow, and score for surgical curability. Am J Med 55:402–414, 1973.

Wilson, HM, Wilson, JP, Slaton, PE, Foster, JH, Liddle, GW, and Hollifield, JW: Saralasin infusion in the recognition of renovascular hypertension. Ann Intern Med 87:36–42, 1977.

Case, DB, Atlas, SA, and Laragh, JH: Position paper: Physiologic effects and diagnostic relevance of acute converting enzyme blockade. In Laragh, JH, Buhler, FR, and Seldin, DW (eds.): Frontiers in Hypertension Research. Springer-Verlag, New York, 1981.

Re, R, Novelline, R, Escourrou, M-T, Athanasoulis, C, Burton, J, and Haber, E: Inhibition of angiotensin-converting enzyme for diagnosis of renal-artery stenosis. N Engl J Med 298:582–586, 1978.

Editorial: Use of saralasin as a diagnostic test in hypertension. Arch Intern Med 142:1437–1440, 1982.

Bookstein, JJ, Abrams, HL, Buenger, RE, Lecky, J, Franklin, SS, Reiss, MD, Bleifer, KH, Klatte, EC, Varady, PD, and Maxwell, MH: Radiologic aspects of renovascular hypertension. Part 2. The role of urography in unilateral renovascular disease. JAMA 220:1225–1230, 1972.

Bookstein, JJ, Abrams, HL, Buenger, RE, Reiss, MD, Lecky, JW, Franklin, SS, Bleifer, KH, Varady, PD, and Maxwell, MH: Radiologic aspects of renovascular hypertension. Part 3. Appraisal of arteriography. JAMA 221:368–374, 1973.

Hillman, BJ, Ovitt, TW, Capp, MP, Prosnitz, EH, Osborne, RW, Jr, Goldstone, J, Zukoski, CF, and Malone, JM: The potential impact of digital video subtraction angiography on screening for renovascular hypertension. Radiol 142:577–579, 1982.

Hypertension of Chronic Renal Failure

Lifschitz, MD: Hypertension in chronic renal failure. In Hypertension. Contemporary Issues in Nephrology, vol. 8. Churchill Livingstone, New York, 1981, pp. 223–246.

Mineralocorticoid-induced Hypertension

Conn, JW: Primary aldosteronism: a new clinical syndrome. J Lab Clin Med 45:6–17, 1955.

Williams, GH: Aldosterone in hypertension. In Hypertension. Contemporary Issues in Nephrology, vol. 8. Churchill Livingstone, New York, 1981, pp. 142–167.

Ferriss, JB, Beevers, DG, Brown, JJ, Davies, DL, Fraser, R, Lever, AF, Mason, P, Neville, AM, and Robertson, JIS: Clinical, biochemical and pathological features of low-renin ("primary") hyperaldosteronism. Am Heart J 95:375–388, 1978.

Weinberger, MH, Grim, CE, Hollifield, JW, Kem, DC, Ganguly, A, Kramer, NJ, Yune, HY, Wellman, H, and Donohue, JP: Primary aldosteronism: diagnosis, localization and treatment. Ann Intern Med 90:386–395, 1979.

Editorial: Glucocorticoid suppressible hyperaldosteronism. A clue to the missing hormone. N Engl J Med 305:1012–1014, 1981.

Bravo, EL, Tarazi, RC, Dustan, HP, Fouad, FM, Textor, SC, Gifford, RW, and Vidt, DG: The changing clinical spectrum of primary aldosteronism. Am J Med 74:641–651, 1983.

Vaughan, NJ, Slater, JDH, Lightman, SL, Jowett, TP, Wiggins, RC, and Ma, JT: The diagnosis of primary hyperaldosteronism. Lancet I:120–126, 1981.

Herf, SM, Teates, DC, Tegtmeyer, CJ, Vaughan, ED, Jr, Ayers, CR, and Carey, RM: Identification and differentiation of surgically correctable hypertension due to primary aldosteronism. Am J Med 67:397–402, 1979.

Streeten, DHP, Tomycz, N, and Anderson, GH: Reliability of screening methods for the diagnosis of primary aldosteronism. Am J Med 67:403–413, 1979.

Ferriss, JB, Brown, JJ, Fraser, R, Kay, AW, Lever, AF, Neville, AM, O'Muircheartaigh, IG, Robertson, JIS, and Symington, T: Hypertension with aldosterone excess and low plasma renin: preoperative distinction between patients with and without adrenocortical tumor. Lancet II:995–1000, 1970.

Davidson, JK, Morley, P, Hurley, GD, and Holford, NGH: Adrenal venography and ultrasound in the investigation of the adrenal gland: an analysis of 58 cases. Br J Radiol 48:435–450, 1975.

Hattery, RR, Sheedy, PF, II, Stephens, DH, and Van Heerden, JA: Computed tomography of the adrenal gland. Seminars Roent 16:290–300, 1981.

Korobkin, M, White, EA, Kressel, HY, Moss, AA, and Montagne, J-P: Computed tomography in the diagnosis of adrenal disease. Am J Roentgenol 132:231–238, 1979.

Dunnick, NR, Doppman, JL, Gill, JR, Jr, Strott, CA, Keiser, HR, and Brennan, MF: Localization of functional adrenal tumors by computed tomography and venous sampling. Radiology 142:429–433, 1982.

Blachley, JD, and Knochel, JP: Tobacco chewer's hypokalemia: licorice revisited. N Engl J Med 302:784–785, 1980.

Ross, EJ, and Linch, DC: Cushing's syndrome—killing disease: discriminatory value of signs and symptoms aiding early diagnosis. Lancet II:646–649, 1982.

Pheochromocytoma

Gittes, RF, and Mahoney, EM: Pheochromocytoma. Urol Clin North Am 4:239–252, 1977.

Goldfien, A: Phaeochromocytoma. Clin Endocrinol Metab 10:607–630, 1981.

Manger, WM, and Gifford, RW, Jr: Pheochromocytoma. Springer-Verlag, New York, 1977.

Bravo, EL: Plasma catecholamines in clinical medicine. Cardiovasc Clin 12:187–196, 1981.

Kaplan, NM, Kramer, NJ, Holland, OB, Sheps, SG, Gomez-Sanchez, C: Single-voided urine metanephrine assays in screening for pheochromocytoma. Arch Intern Med 137:190–193, 1977.

Stewart, BH, Bravo, EL, Haaga, J, Meaney, TF, Tarazi, R: Localization of pheochromocytoma by computed tomography. N Engl J Med 299:460–461, 1978.

Bravo, EL, Tarazi, RC, Fouad, FM, Vidt, DG, and Gifford, RW, Jr: Clonidine-suppression test. A useful aid in the diagnosis of pheochromocytoma. N Engl J Med 305:623–626, 1981.

Estafanous, FG, and Tarazi, RC: Systemic arterial hypertension associated with cardiac surgery. Am J Cardiol 46:685–694, 1980.

Atuk, NO: Pheochromocytoma: diagnosis, localization, and treatment. Hosp Prac 18(April):187–202, 1983.

Kadir, S, and Robinette, C: Accuracy of angiography in the localization of pheochromocytoma. J Urol 126:789–793, 1981.

4

DIAGNOSTIC WORK-UP OF THE HYPERTENSIVE PATIENT

The laboratory evaluation of patients with hypertension is a subject of debate. Although no one recommends treatment without any work-up or laboratory tests, many patients are being treated without even a minimum evaluation. On the other hand, the work-up is often overdone, and on this point, the following quotation by the respected authority Dr. Edward D. Freis is very apropos.

Unfortunately, medical tradition has grossly exaggerated the importance of detecting *curable* hypertension. For years, physicians have been taught that their major obligation was to rule out curable hypertension, and once this was done, their obligation to the patient has been discharged. The physician's responsibility only begins with the ruling out of curable hypertension, and he must not strain unduly his own or the patient's resources in doing so. The problem is to restore a perspective which is consonant with the relative worth of diagnostic and therapeutic procedures that are most apt to be effective in preventing the major complications of hypertension. The greatest cost-benefit ratio lies in the treatment, specifically in the drug treatment, of hypertension.

The majority of investigators and clinicians expert in the care of hypertensive patients now believe that the routine laboratory work-up of a patient *should be relatively limited.* Practically everyone agrees that the laboratory evaluation should focus on defining the patient's degree of target organ damage, if any, and searching for curable causes of hypertension that are suggested by the clinical presentation. If the patient's history and physical examination have provided no important clues suggestive of secondary hypertension (see Chapter 3), the small number of essential tests to be ordered before the initiation of antihypertensive therapy *can be restricted.* Table 4–1 summarizes the approach of differing segments of the clinical community, ranging from a group of practicing internists in Atlanta, Georgia, to the recommendations of the Task Force of The National High Blood Pressure Education Program. As can be seen, all agree on obtaining a urinalysis, serum potassium, blood urea nitrogen (BUN) or creatinine, blood glucose, cholesterol, and resting ECG. Although the Task

TABLE 4–1. RECOMMENDED MINIMUM WORK-UP FOR HYPERTENSIVES

	Six practicing internists, Atlanta, 1976	Task Force I, National High Blood Pressure Education Program	Inter-Society Commission for Heart Disease Resources	Recognized authorities**
History	Yes	Yes	Yes	Yes
Physical	Yes	Yes	Yes	Yes
CBC or Hct	Yes	No	Yes	Yes
Urinalysis	Yes	Yes	Yes	Yes
Serum potassium	Yes	Yes	Yes	Yes
BUN or creatinine	Yes	Yes	Yes	Yes
Blood glucose	Yes	Yes	Yes	Yes
Uric acid	Yes	"Helpful"	Yes	Yes
Cholesterol	Yes	Yes	Yes	Yes
Resting ECG	Yes	Yes	Yes	Yes
Chest x-ray	Yes	"Helpful"	Yes	Yes
IV urogram	Yes (1) No (5)	No	No	Yes (3)[A] No (8)
VMA or metanephrine	Yes (1) No (5)	No	No	Yes (2)[B] No (9)
Sedimentation rate	Yes	No	No	No
Peripheral plasma renin assay	No	No	No	Yes (3)[A] No (8)
24-hour urine sodium	No	No	No	Yes (2)[C] No (9)
Serum calcium	Yes*	No	No	Yes (1)[D] No (10)

*All six internists would order automated battery of 18 blood chemistries.
**Dustan, Freis, Finnerty, Gifford, Gunnells, Hunt, Laragh, Maxwell, Moser, Oparil, and Williams.
A = Hunt, Maxwell, Oparil; B = Hunt, Maxwell; C = Hunt, Oparil; D = Hunt (in a personal communication Hunt emphasizes that he varies his "minimal work-up" depending on the severity of the hypertension and the level of the diastolic blood pressure).

Modified From Wilber, JA: Cardiovasc Med, Jan. 1977

Force designated the chest x-ray and uric acid as "helpful," we believe they should be performed routinely. The purpose of these tests is to (a) look for unsuspected evidence of a curable cause of hypertension, (b) determine the presence and degree of end-organ damage, and (c) determine whether other common conditions statistically shown to be more common in the hypertensive population, such as diabetes, hyperuricemia, or hypercalcemia, are present. Obviously, the value of some of these tests often overlaps these categories.

In terms of an indication of a curable cause of hypertension, the most helpful finding from the laboratory tests listed in Table 4–1 is spontaneous hypokalemia, i.e., hypokalemia unprovoked by diuretic administration. A further discussion of the importance of unprovoked hypokalemia can be found in Chapter 3. Much less commonly observed clues for secondary hypertension include rib notching on the chest x-ray (coarctation of aorta). Of course, an elevated level of BUN or creatinine might indicate either renal insufficiency resulting from long-standing hypertension or hypertension resulting from acute or chronic renal failure (see Chapter 3 for extensive discussion of curable hypertension). Refractoriness to appropriate pharmacologic therapy may be a clue to secondary hypertension, particularly renovascular hypertension. Likewise, a sudden unexplained increase in blood pressure should raise the suspicion that a superimposed condition such as renal artery stenosis has occurred.

We favor the measurement of serum calcium concentration before the initiation of pharmacologic therapy. The principal value of this determination lies in providing a baseline for subsequent comparison should the serum calcium concentration be elevated in the course of diuretic therapy. Rarely, the pretreatment serum calcium level may be elevated, and since hypercalcemia per se tends to increase the blood pressure, it may be responsible in part for the elevated blood pressure, in addition to signaling the presence of an important disorder.

Finally, a major and often forgotten component of the work-up is patient education. A major effort should be made to inform the patient fully of his condition, his risk, and the indefinitely prolonged need for therapy. Because they are not trained in health education, physicians are often reluctant to spend the considerable amount of time required for appropriate patient education. Unfortunately, if this step is omitted or given only cursory attention, other efforts may be wasted.

Laboratory Data Helpful During the Course of Antihypertensive Therapy

These tests are essentially the same as those ordered in the pretherapy evaluation of a patient with hypertension (Table 4–1). Their purpose is to (a) facilitate assessment of possible complications of therapy and (b) anticipate progression or improvement of end-organ dysfunction.

For example, the potential side effects of diuretics subtend a wide array of potential laboratory abnormalities, including hypokalemia, dilutional hyponatremia, hypochloremic metabolic alkalosis, hyperglycemia, azotemia, hyperuricemia, hypercalcemia, hypophosphatemia, hypomagnesemia, and rarely neutropenia or thrombocytopenia. Similarly, certain medications can produce impairment of hepatic function. For example, methyldopa administration may be associated with an increase in SGOT levels, and prolonged use of hydralazine at high doses can induce an ANA-positive, systemic lupus erythematosus–like syndrome. The specific side effects of the various antihypertensive agents and the variable need for laboratory surveillance in the use of these drugs are considered in detail in Chapter 6.

REFERENCES

Wilber JA: The minimum work-up for hypertension. Cardiovasc Med, pp. 55–64, Jan. 1977.

Epstein, M: The role of renin measurements in the management of hypertension. The Kidney *10*:1–6, Jan. 1977.

Ferguson, RK: Cost and yield of the hypertensive evaluation. Ann Intern Med *82*:761–765, 1975.

Mentser, M: Diagnosis and treatment of hypertension in children. Pediatr Clin North Am *29*:933–945, 1982.

Bartter, FC: Renin-aldosterone profiling in hypertension. Ann Intern Med *87*:596–612, 1977.

Gavras, H., and Gavras, I.: The renin-angiotensin system. *In* Hypertension. Contemporary Issues in Nephrology, vol. 8. Churchill Livingstone, New York, 1981, pp. 65–99.

Henzl, MR: Natural and synthetic female sex hormones. *In* Yen, SSC, and Jaffee, RB (eds.): Reproductive Endocrinology: Physiology, Pathophysiology, and Clinical Management. WB Saunders Co., Philadelphia, 1978, pp. 421–468.

II

Principles of Management

The risk of untreated hypertension and the benefits of effective management having been considered, this section will examine strategies of management of hypertensive disease. Initially, we will consider the larger issue of the management of patients with primary hypertension without renal insufficiency or other major complications. Afterward, the treatment of secondary and complicated forms of hypertension will be examined.

TABLE 5–1. GOALS OF ANTIHYPERTENSIVE THERAPY

1. Reduce diastolic pressure to at least 90 mm Hg.
2. Reduce diastolic pressure to lowest level consistent with safety and tolerance.
3. In patient with moderate or severe or resistant hypertension attempt to normalize pressure; lesser control, however, may be acceptable.
4. In patient with complicated hypertension try to improve organ function (or prevent further deterioration).
   a. Obviate congestive heart failure.
   b. Prevent end-stage renal failure.
   c. Prevent additional cerebrovascular accidents.

Goals of Therapy (Table 5–1)

The 1980 report of the Joint National Committee on Detection, Evaluation, and Treatment of High Blood Pressure stressed the 'importance of establishing a therapeutic goal for the individual patient. It further stated that the initial goal should be to achieve and maintain diastolic blood pressures at less than 90 mm Hg with a further goal of reaching the lowest diastolic pressure consistent with patient acceptability and potential toxicity. Although, because of side effects, a lesser degree of control may have to be accepted in patients with moderate to severe hypertension, near normotension can often be established if the patient is compliant and the physician persistent in his search for the proper medication and dosages. Fortunately, partial control has also been shown to reduce cardiovascular morbidity. In the patient with complicated hypertension, the goals should be as above. In addition, however, the plan should be to preserve end-organ function, for example, to maintain renal function in the patient with renal insufficiency and to obviate congestive heart failure in the patient with hypertensive cardiovascular disease.

5

NONDRUG TREATMENT OF HYPERTENSION

Although most of the emphasis on treating hypertension has been in the use of antihypertensive drugs, it should be pointed out that there are several nondrug therapies available for the management of hypertensive patients. In patients with mild hypertension (diastolic blood pressure 95 to 100 mm Hg), nondrug therapy alone often provides adequate control of the blood pressure, so that drug therapy may be unneeded or at least postponed. In those patients who need pharmacologic intervention, nondrug therapy may constitute an adjunct. This may reduce the dose requirement of medications, potentiate their good effects, and diminish their side effects.

TYPES OF NONDRUG THERAPY

Table 5–2 lists the major available nondrug therapeutic modalities. These include weight reduction, sodium restriction, exercise, and behavior-modifying techniques.

Weight Reduction

Weight gain is often associated with an increase in blood pressure, and weight loss with a fall. The relation between obesity and blood pressure is particularly strong in children, and there is hope for prevention of future hypertension by prevention of childhood obesity.

The best demonstration that weight will lower the blood pressure has come from Israel. Of 81 hypertensives who participated in a four-month diet and lost an average of 9.5 kg, 79 had a statistically significant fall in blood pressure, averaging about 30/20 mm Hg. The frequent failure of diets to maintain weight loss renders it unlikely that many obese hypertensives will achieve long-term control by weight reduction alone. Nevertheless, we should try to correct obesity in hypertensive patients. Ideally, this should be accomplished before antihypertensive drug therapy is begun; the hope for control of hypertension may motivate the patient to start a diet, and the decline in pressure may provide positive reinforcement to keep the patient on the diet. On the other

TABLE 5–2.   NONDRUG TREATMENT OF HYPERTENSION

1. Weight reduction
2. Exercise
3. Dietary sodium restriction
4. Transcendental meditation
5. Biofeedback

hand, it is inappropriate to withhold pharmacologic therapy while waiting expectantly for the effects of a weight loss that may not be forthcoming. Instead, if the blood pressure appears to be well controlled, an attempt to withdraw antihypertensive medications can be made after the weight loss has occurred.

Exercise

The role of exercise in the routine treatment of hypertension is controversial. Although there is some evidence that a regular program of isotonic or dynamic exercise may lower the blood pressure, the available evidence is skimpy and poorly controlled. Some studies in human subjects have suggested that regular physical activity lowers blood pressure, but in a recent review of cardiovascular adaptations to training, the available data were not believed to support this conclusion. Although some of the aforementioned studies are promising, the place of regular exercise in routine antihypertensive therapy cannot be determined as yet.

In contrast to isotonic exercise, isometric or static exercise provides no benefit to the hypertensive patient. In fact, the marked rise in both systolic and diastolic pressures that occurs during isometric contractions occasionally precipitates vascular catastrophes. Therefore, patients with severe hypertension should be advised to avoid isometric exercise, such as carrying a heavy suitcase.

Sodium Restriction

As noted earlier, excessive intake of sodium is a likely contributing factor to the development of hypertension. A reduction of dietary sodium intake may help lower an elevated pressure. With proper instruction and encouragement, most hypertensives will follow a diet moderately restricted in sodium. By reducing the usual daily intake from 150 to 200 mEq to 75 to 100 mEq, patients may achieve a significant fall in blood pressure. Even though the encountered decrease will not normalize the blood pressure in patients with moderate to advanced hypertension, and the fall is not predictable, sodium restriction may eliminate the need for, or reduce the dose required of, other antihypertensive medications.

Before embarking on a review of dietary sodium restriction, it is worthwhile to consider the sodium requirements for healthy adults and the range of sodium intake in the typical American diet. It should be underscored that in the absence of unusual losses, such as from diarrhea, the body needs for sodium are exceedingly small. The Food and Nutrition Board of the National Academy of Sciences–National Research Council considers that daily intakes of 1.1 to 3.3 g of sodium are adequate for the healthy adult.

Most dietary sodium is found in the form of sodium chloride (table salt), which is approximately 40 per cent sodium and 60 per cent chloride. One teaspoon of salt contains approximately 2.0 g of sodium (87 mEq). The daily sodium intake of adult Americans is estimated to range between 2.3 and 6.9 g of sodium (about 1 to 3 teaspoons, or 6 to 17 g, of salt).

Various sources express dietary sodium content in milliequivalents of sodium or in grams or milligrams of either salt or sodium. Not only can this be quite confusing to the clinician, it sometimes leads to regrettable mistakes—there is about 2½ times as much sodium in a gram of sodium (43 mEq) as in a gram of salt (17 mEq). Table 5–3 presents a brief summary of how to convert these units.

One may ask why compliance with dietary sodium restriction is so poor. One reason is that the physician is fighting an uphill battle against custom and firmly established habits. Our eating habits have changed greatly since World War II. Convenience foods and fast-food restaurants and take-out services have become a way of life for our mobile society. Unfortunately, convenience and processed foods contain much more sodium and fat, usually saturated fat, and fast-food items entail a very high calorie intake. Finally, a caveat is warranted regarding salt content of the so-called ethnic foods. Although these foods often contain an incredible amount of salt, one needs to exercise some degree of restraint in proscribing all such foods. The physician must have some degree of cultural sensitivity when recommending alterations in eating habits in his pursuit of lower blood pressure.

Another major deterrent to successful dietary sodium restriction is the lack of awareness both by patients and even by some physicians of the sodium content of food. As noted in Appendix 1, in addition to the salt we knowingly sprinkle on our food, some commonly consumed foods that are not salty to the palate contain large amounts of sodium. This is particularly true of processed food. As an example, although a tomato contains merely 14 mg of sodium a cup of tomato soup contains 932 mg. Similarly, an English muffin contains approximately 300 mg of sodium. Salted or brined meats and fish are obviously higher in salt content than the uncured forms. Many canned vegetables are packed in a salt solution or brine.

Frozen vegetables are usually processed without added salt. However, starchy vegetables like lima beans and peas are frequently sorted in brine before freezing. Frozen vegetables with added sauces, mushrooms, or nuts are higher in sodium than the plain varieties.

TABLE 5–3. SALT AND SODIUM CONVERSIONS

Sodium to salt (NaCl) equivalent	Milligrams of sodium content ÷ .40 = milligrams of salt
Salt to sodium	Milligrams of salt × .40 = milligrams of sodium
Sodium in milligrams to sodium in milliequivalents	Milligrams of sodium ÷ 23 (atomic weight of sodium) = milliequivalents of sodium
Milliequivalents of sodium to milligrams of sodium	Milliequivalents of sodium × 23 = milligrams of sodium

Canned and frozen fruits are not usually processed with added salt, but some companies add small amounts of salt to prevent darkening of some fruits and to enhance the flavor of applesauce. Some canned and frozen fruits, and most canned whole tomatoes, are dipped in sodium hydroxide so that they can be easily peeled. This process causes these foods to have higher sodium levels than are found in the fresh food. Canned and bottled citrus drinks are sometimes buffered with sodium citrate. Some popular flavoring agents high in sodium are soy sauce, Worcestershire sauce, catsup, pickles, olives, and garlic, onion, and celery salts. Sodium ion exchange is used in processing some wines to reduce sediment and clarify the product.

Chemical ingredients that contain sodium may be added during food processing. Some examples of these ingredients are monosodium glutamate, or MSG (a flavor enhancer); sodium saccharin (a sweetener); sodium phosphates (emulsifiers, stabilizers, buffers); sodium citrate (a buffer); sodium caseinate (a thickener and binder); and sodium benzoate and sodium nitrite (preservatives). Finally, household staples like baking powder and baking soda are sodium compounds.

When salt is taken away from patients placed on a sodium-restricted diet, they often complain that their food tastes "flat." Nevertheless, it must be emphasized that adopting a low-salt diet does not necessarily relegate the patient to a bland, boring, and repetitive diet. With the recent increased emphasis on sodium and the deleterious effects of high sodium intake, ingenious low-salt recipes have proliferated and now appear routinely in newspapers and women's magazines. Special cookbooks exist to meet all pocketbooks, if not all palates. The emphasis of most is that there is more to low-salt life than just discarding the salt shaker. Seasoning can be substituted for salt. Angostura bitters, cumin, vinegar, vermouth, and table wine (cooking wine contains salt) have all done much to enhance low-salt diets. Spices, herbs, and lemon juice may not only replace salt, but may complement and enhance the natural flavor of many foods.

So-called salt substitutes usually contain potassium instead of sodium and should be used only on the advice of a physician. In addition, since some substitutes produce a bitter taste when used during cooking, they should generally be added just before serving.

Appendix 2 provides a compilation of specific suggestions for the flavoring, without salt, of several common foods.

One of the most down-to-earth low-salt cookbooks is the American Heart Association book *Cooking Without Your Salt Shaker*. Craig Claiborne's *Gourmet Diet Book* and Eleanor Brenner's *Gourmet Cooking Without Salt* are probably the most sophisticated guides currently available. These provide recipes for such foods as low-salt pâtés and exotica like the eggplant delicacy Baba Ghanouju.

It is imperative that the physician not merely hand the patient a standard diet sheet listing a 2-gram or 90-mEq sodium diet. If this is done, it is likely that compliance, and perhaps even the patient, will be lost. One of the biggest problems in patient compliance is that if the patient is merely handed a standard printed diet regimen, the impression is conveyed that the diet is not an important factor in therapy. And if the patient feels that the physician does not really think the diet is important, it will not be important to him either.

It is worse yet to overrestrict the patient with a needlessly severe 1-gram sodium diet, hoping he will reduce his sodium at least to 2 grams. In such a case the patient cannot help becoming very negative. But if the physician has a positive approach to dietary control, and if he makes the diet an important part of therapy, then the patient is more likely to follow it.

When giving the diet prescription to the patient, saying something negative, like, "I don't know how well you can follow this," or, "Do the best you can," or, "This may not help you very much," may result in losing the patient. It makes a world of difference to say something positive, like, "This is going to be good for you," "This is going to help you do this or that," or "My wife can do this, I can do it, you can do it."

Finally, implicit in our comments is the fact the sole burden for prescribing and explaining the low-salt diet should not fall solely on the shoulders of the clinician. A motivated and experienced dietician should be an integral part of the management team. Nevertheless, the clinician must have a feel for the recommendations of the dietician and be in a position to comment on, clarify, and reinforce them.

It is important to emphasize that moderate sodium restriction not only tends to facilitate a fall in blood pressure, but also serves to lessen the loss of potassium induced by diuretics. The mechanism for this phenomenon is presumed to be a decrease in the delivery of sodium to the distal nephron site at which potassium is secreted. A carefully performed study has indicated that diuretic-induced potassium loss may be halved by concomitant reduction in dietary sodium intake.

Interesting preliminary evidence is beginning to accumulate regarding the potentially beneficial effect of an increased dietary potassium-sodium ratio. Thus, it appears that increasing the intake of potassium, independent of any decrease in that of sodium, has blood pressure–lowering properties. The mechanism for this phenomenon is unknown, and more investigation is needed to substantiate the early favorable results.

Behavioral Methods

The assumption that increased central nervous system sympathetic activity is an etiologic factor in the development and maintenance of essential hypertension constitutes the basis for behavioral treatment. Presumably, if one could modify the central nervous system response to stress, blood pressure could be reduced.

Behavioral therapy attempts to modify this response by taking advantage of two observations. The first is that human subjects can voluntarily induce a hypometabolic state of decreased sympathetic arousal in which heart rate, oxygen consumption, respiratory rate, blood lactate concentration, carbon dioxide elimination, and blood pressure can be reduced. The ability to achieve this state of relaxation, perhaps the opposite of the fight or flight response, can be learned and is the rationale for transcendental meditation, hypnosis, yoga, and recently developed noncultic "relaxation response." The second observation is that human subjects and animals can learn to control voluntarily the functions of the autonomic nervous system, including blood pressure. Apparatus have been developed that can give heartbeat-to-heartbeat information (feedback) on the level of blood pressure, which can help to train a subject to control it. This is the basis for biofeedback therapy for hypertension.

Biofeedback. Biofeedback uses modern technology to provide visual or auditory signals of a precise level to the subject. Both animals and humans can be trained to recognize the level of pressure and to raise and lower systolic and diastolic pressure voluntarily, probably by regulation of peripheral vascular resistance.

Although it has been clearly shown that biofeedback can modestly lower blood pressure for brief periods in normotensive subjects, it has seldom been used alone as therapy for hypertension. In the few studies published on small groups of patients, reduction of blood pressure by as much as 18/8 mm Hg has been achieved. Others have reported much less improvement.

REFERENCES

Alderman, MH: Position paper. The variation in risk among hypertensive patients: Is broad scale therapy to help only a few justifiable? What pressure levels should be treated? *In* Laragh, JH, et al.: Frontiers in Hypertension Research. Springer-Verlag, New York, 1981, pp. 9–14.

Editorial: Lowering blood pressure without drugs. Lancet II: 459–461, 1980.

Stamler, J, Farinaro, E, Mojonnier, LM, Hall, Y, Moss, D, and Stamler, R: Prevention and control of hypertension by nutritional-hygienic means. JAMA 243:1819–1823, 1980.

The Joint Committee on Detection, Evaluation, and Treatment of High Blood Pressure. The 1980 report of the Joint National Committee on Detection, Evaluation, and Treatment of High Blood Pressure. Arch Intern Med, 140:1280–1285, 1980.

Weight Reduction

Reisin, E, Able, R, and Modan, M: Effect of weight loss without salt restriction in the reduction of blood pressure in overweight hypertensive patients. N Engl J Med 298:1–6, 1978.

Tobian, L: Hypertension and obesity. N Engl J Med 298:46–47, 1978.

Sims, EAH, and Berchtold, P: Obesity and hypertension. Mechanisms and implications for management. JAMA 247:49–52, 1982.

Turk, ML, Sowers, J, Dornfeld, L, Kledzik, G, and Maxwell, M: The effect of weight reduction on blood pressure, plasma renin activity, and plasma aldosterone levels in obese patients. N Engl J Med 304:903–933, 1981.

Puska, P, Iacono, JM, Nissinen, A, Korhomen, HJ, Vartiainen, E, Pietinem, P, Dougherty, R, Leino, U, Mutanen, M, Moisio, S, and Huttunen, J: Controlled, randomized trial of the effect of dietary fat on blood pressure. Lancet I:1–10, 1983.

Exercise

Björntorp, P: Hypertension and exercise. Hypertension 4(Suppl. III): 56–59, 1982.

Dietary Sodium Restriction

Morgan, T, Adams, W, Gillies, A, Wilson, M, Morgan G, and Carney, S: Hypertension treated by salt restriction. Lancet I: 227–230, 1978.

Ram, CV, Garrett, BN, and Kaplan, NM: Moderate sodium restriction and various diuretics in the treatment of hypertension. Arch Intern Med 141:1015–1019, 1981.

Miles, JM, and Miles TS: Effect of processed foods on the salt intake of preschool children. Med J Aust II: 23–25, 1982.

Kaplan, NM, Simmons, M, McPhee, C, Carnegie, A, Stefanu, C, and Cade, S: Two techniques to improve adherence to dietary sodium restriction in the treatment of hypertension. Arch Intern Med 142:1639–1641, 1982.

Paul, AA, and Southgate, DAT: McCance and Widdowson's The Composition of Foods, 4th ed. Her Majesty's Stationery Office, London, 1976.

Mayo Clinic: Mayo Clinic Diet Manual, 5th ed. (Edited by Pemberton, CM, and Gastineau, CF.) W. B. Saunders Co., Philadelphia, 1981.

Meneely, GR, and Battarbee, HD: High sodium–low potassium environment and hypertension. Am J Cardiol 38:768–785, 1976.

Dietary Alterations Other than for Sodium

MacGregor, GA, Smith, SJ, Markandu, ND, Banks, RA, and Sagnella, GA: Moderate potassium supplementation in essential hypertension. Lancet II: 567–570, 1982.

MacGregor, GA: Dietary sodium and potassium intake and blood pressure. Lancet I:750–753, 1983.

Henningsen, NC, Larsson, L, and Nelson, D: Hypertension, potassium and the kitchen. Lancet I:133, 1983.

Belizan, JM, Villar, J, Pineda, O, Gonzalez, AE, Sainz, E, Garrera, G, and Sibrian, R: Reduction of blood pressure with calcium supplementation in young adults. JAMA 249:1161–1165, 1983.

McCarron, DA: Calcium, magnesium, and phosphorus balance in human and experimental hypertension. Hypertension 4(Suppl. III):27–33, 1982.

Frankel, BL, Patel, DJ, Horwitz, D, Freidewald, WT, and Gaardner, KR: Treatment of hypertension with biofeedback and relaxation techniques. Psychosom Med 40:276–293, 1978.

6

PHARMACOLOGIC MANAGEMENT OF HYPERTENSION

Sometimes the clinician is bewildered by the myriad of marketed antihypertensive agents. As an example, half of the antihypertensive drugs used today were not available 10 years ago, and many additional new agents are currently under investigation. Newer drugs are frequently far more effective and versatile than the ones they supplant.

Ideally, the underlying cause of a patient's hypertension would be identified, and this identification would be followed by prescription of specific therapy. Unfortunately, except in the case of pheochromocytoma, certain instances of drug-induced hypertension, and clear-cut hypervolemia (as in terminal renal failure), this is rarely possible.

In practice, an empiric experience-proven Step-Care method is employed. In patients with moderate to severe hypertension, combinations of drugs acting at different sites are used. This permits blunting of unwanted reflex responses to certain drugs, reduces the intolerable side effects that may be encountered when large doses of single drugs are given, and allows rational therapeutic regimens to be tailored to individual patients.

A practical schema of drug classification is helpful in understanding the mechanism of action of antihypertensive agents and their place in the therapy of the individual patient. We favor a classification based upon site of action. The various medications can then be grouped as diuretics, inhibitors of the sympathetic nervous system (either peripherally or centrally acting), arteriolar vasodilators, inhibitors of the renin-angiotensin-aldosterone axis, or calcium entry blockers.

Sites of Action of Antihypertensive Drugs

Figure 6–1 depicts in a schematic fashion the possible sites of action of various blood pressure–lowering drugs. Irrespective of the underlying cause of hypertension, these medications reduce pressure by an effect on one or a number of mechanisms that modulate circulatory homeostasis. Thus, antihypertensive properties are shared by sympatholytic agents that act centrally or peripherally to diminish sympathetic tone; by beta-blockers or diuretics that

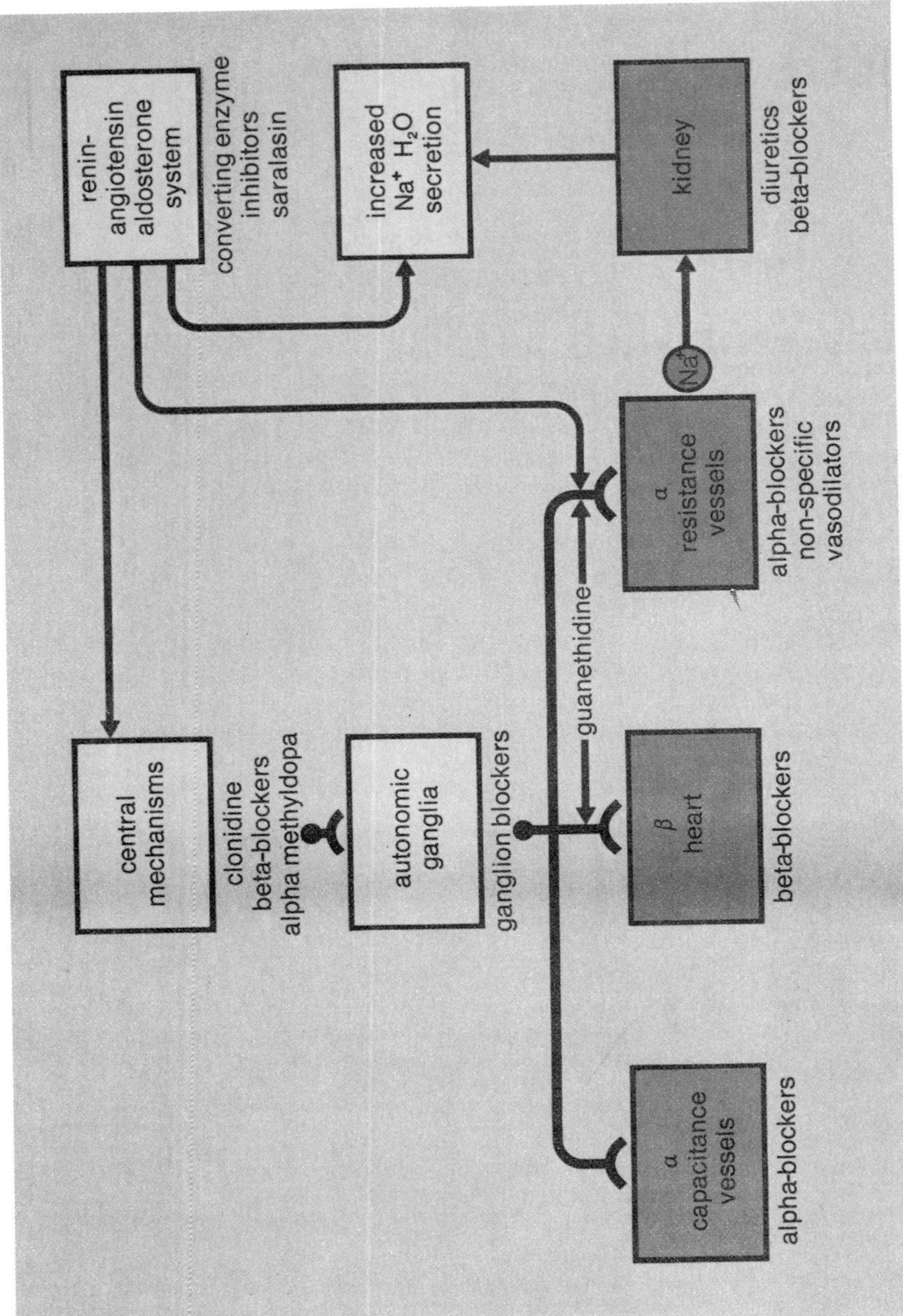

FIGURE 6–1. Possible sites of action of various blood pressure–lowering drugs. Irrespective of the underlying cause of hypertension, these medications reduce pressure by an effect on one or a number of mechanisms that modulate circulatory homeostasis. Thus, antihypertensive properties are shared by sympatholytic agents that act centrally or peripherally to diminish sympathetic tone; by beta-blockers or diuretics that reduce cardiac output by decreasing the heart rate or extracellular fluid volume, respectively; by agents that inhibit the activity of the renin-angiotensin system; and finally by drugs that by diverse mechanisms produce arteriolar smooth muscle dilation. (Reproduced from Hypertension Illustrated by WS Peart, PS Sever, JD Swales, and R Tarazi, courtesy of Gower Medical Publishing.)

reduce cardiac output by decreasing the heart rate or extracellular fluid volume, respectively; by agents that inhibit the activity of the renin-angiotensin system; and finally by drugs that by diverse mechanisms produce arteriolar smooth muscle dilation. The latter may be through nonspecific relaxation of smooth muscle, either by an alteration in the properties of the blood vessel wall (reducing the salt and water content [diuretics]) or by antagonism of the entry of calcium into smooth muscle cells (calcium entry blockers).

Overview of the Adrenergic Nervous System

Before proceeding to discuss specific medications, it will be helpful to review briefly some aspects of the adrenergic nervous system. This will permit the reader to appreciate better the hemodynamic and the adverse effects of the alpha- and beta-blocking agents that constitute a major segment of our antihypertensive armamentarium.

Figure 6–2 schematically depicts the types of alpha receptors located at the terminals of adrenergic neurons. The designations *presynaptic* and *postsynaptic* are morphologic and based on whether the receptors lie on the neuronal or the distal side of the synaptic cleft. Conversely, the designations *alpha-1* and *alpha-2* are based on the response to various agonists and antagonists. Although subtypes 1 and 2 may be present at both presynaptic and postsynaptic sites, the alpha-1 receptor has been considered to predominate at postsynaptic sites and the alpha-2 receptor at the presynaptic locations.

As can be seen in Figures 6–3 and 6–4, the transmission of an impulse to the nerve terminal results in the release of norepinephrine. This neurotransmitter crosses from the presynaptic to the postsynaptic vascular smooth muscle side of the synaptic cleft and causes vasoconstriction by stimulating the postsynaptic receptor. Some of the norepinephrine released by the neuron also interacts with presynaptic receptors (Fig. 6–3). This activates a negative (inhibitory) feedback-loop that tends to prevent excessive release of norepinephrine.

Furthermore, although controversial, it is believed that alteration of alpha receptor activity within the central nervous system accounts, at least in part, for the action of certain sympatholytic agents such as clonidine. Thus, it has been suggested that clonidine stimulates central alpha-2 receptors. This would lead to a diminished outflow of sympathetic impulses from the central nervous system, eventuating in decreased vascular tone.

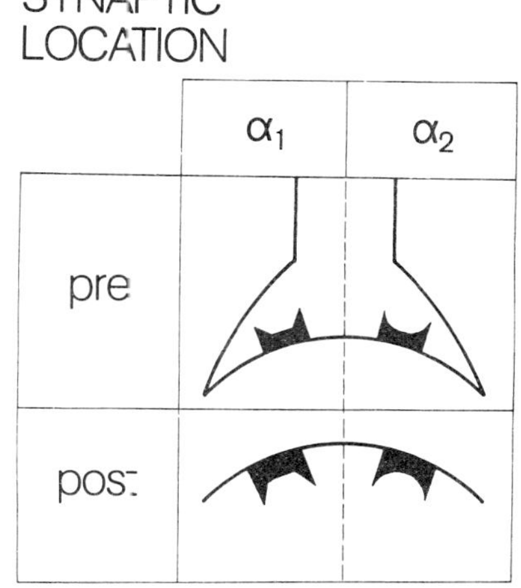

FIGURE 6–2. Types of alpha receptors located at the terminals of adrenergic neurons. The designations *presynaptic* and *postsynaptic* are morphologic and based on whether the receptors lie on the neuronal or the distal side of the synaptic cleft. Conversely, the designations *alpha-1* and *alpha-2* are based on the response to various agonists and antagonists. Although subtypes 1 and 2 may be present at both presynaptic and postsynaptic sites, the alpha-1 receptor has been considered to predominate at postsynaptic sites and the alpha-2 receptor at the presynaptic locations. (Reproduced with permission from Kobinger, W: Chest 83:297, 1983.)

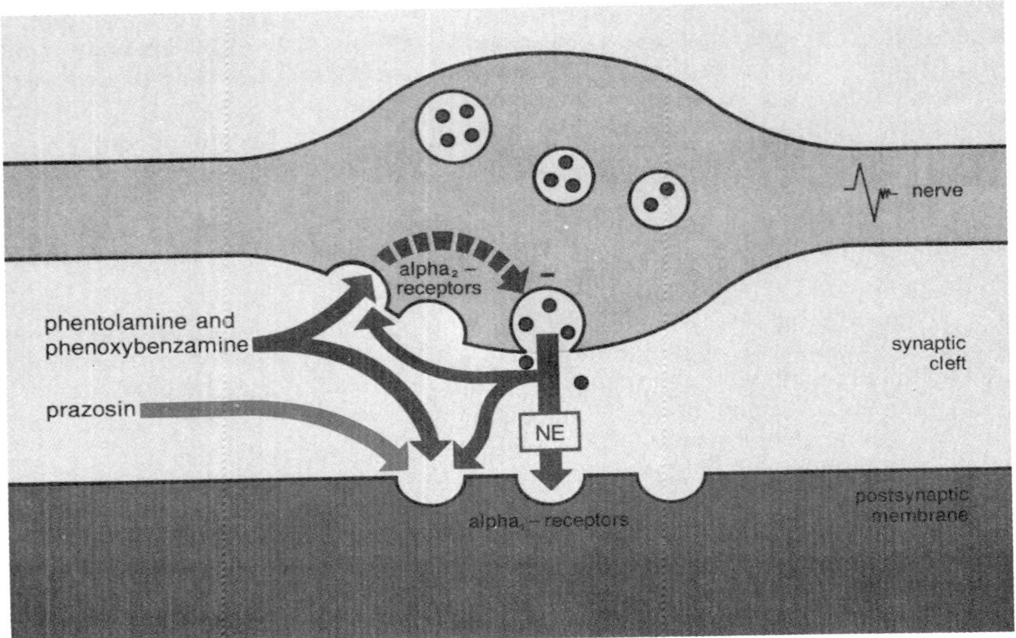

FIGURE 6–3. Sites of action of alpha-blocking drugs on presynaptic and postsynaptic receptors. As can be seen, the transmission of an impulse to the nerve terminal results in the release of norepinephrine (*NE*). This neurotransmitter crosses from the presynaptic to the postsynaptic vascular smooth muscle side of the synaptic cleft and causes vasoconstriction by stimulating the postsynaptic (predominantly alpha-1) receptor. Some of the norepinephrine released by the neuron also interacts with presynaptic (predominantly alpha-2) receptors. This activates a negative (inhibitory) feedback-loop that tends to prevent excessive release of norepinephrine. Whereas phentolamine and phenoxybenzamine nonselectively antagonize both the presynaptic and postsynaptic receptors, prazosin predominately inhibits the postsynaptic (alpha-1) receptor. (Reproduced from Hypertension Illustrated by WS Peart, PS Sever, JD Swales, and R Tarazi, courtesy of Gower Medical Publishing.)

Finally, Figure 6–4 also depicts an interrelation between the beta and alpha adrenergic systems that might be of considerable importance. As illustrated, the nerve terminal contains beta receptors whose stimulation promotes norepinephrine release. Thus, beta-blockers might act in part by reducing vasoconstriction (and therefore peripheral resistance) through indirect inhibition of the alpha adrenergic system.

Step-Care

The prototypical approach for the pharmacologic management of hypertension is the so-called Step-Care method, which has been the recommendation of the Joint National Committee on Detection, Evaluation, and Treatment of High Blood Pressure, both in 1977 and in 1980. Figure 6–5 depicts the algorithm of Step-Care.

If nonpharmacologic means fail to control hypertension, Step-1 consists of the initiation of diuretic therapy. If the use of diuretics does not suffice, Step-2 consists of the addition of an inhibitor of the sympathetic nervous system. Likewise, in a patient whose hypertension is not controlled by diuretic plus a sympathetic inhibitor, Step-3, the further addition of a vasodilator, is undertaken. Finally, in the small percentage of patients resistant to such a triple-drug regimen, the clinician employs Step-4, which means the addition or substitution of one of the very potent agents such as minoxidil, captopril, or

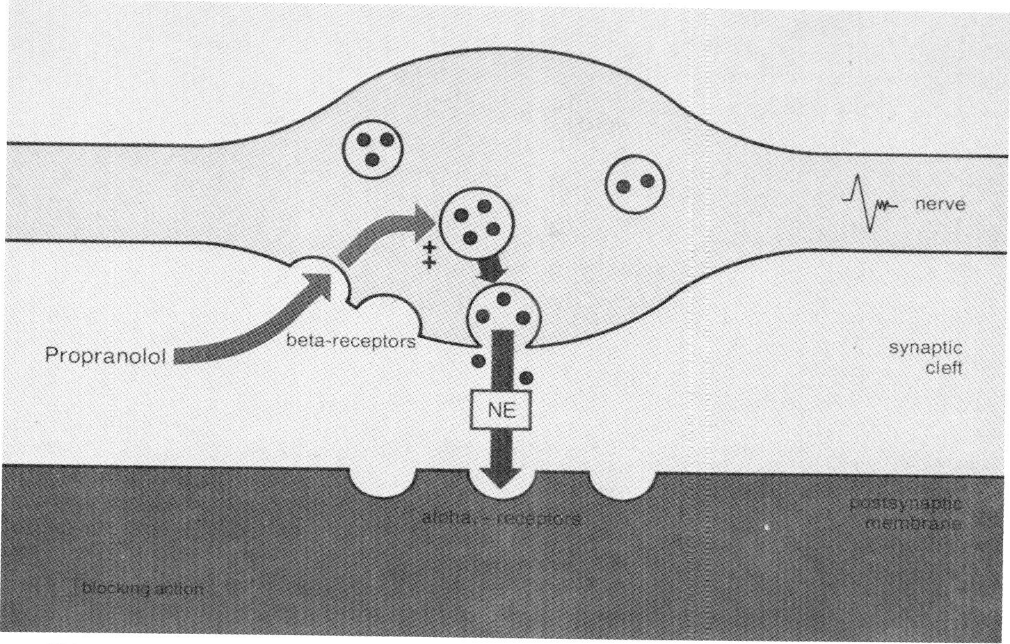

FIGURE 6–4. Peripheral sympathetic nerve terminal demonstrating the putative presynaptic beta-adrenergic receptor. Stimulation of this receptor has been postulated to lead to an inhibition of norepinephrine (*NE*) release. (Reproduced from Hypertension Illustrated by WS Peart, PS Sever, JD Swales, and R Tarazi, courtesy of Gower Medical Publishing.)

guanethidine. Within each Step, the dosages of newly added agents are gradually and carefully titrated upward in relation to the blood pressure and the appearance of side effects.

This algorithmic plan has the advantage of simplicity, logic, and efficacy proven by an enormous clinical experience. Although we agree with its use as a basic modus operandi, it is not necessarily the only reasonable approach to the management of hypertensive patients. As an example, the reader is referred to our discussion of the choice of a Step-1 agent and the role of nondiuretic monotherapy (see Chapter 8).

STEP-CARE APPROACH TO THE MANAGEMENT OF HYPERTENSION

4	Use of one of the more potent agents (e.g. minoxidil), or addition of a second Step 2 agent.
3	Vasodilator
2	Inhibitor of the sympathetic nervous system (β-blocker, clonidine, methyldopa, etc.) — Thiazide-type diuretic
1	Thiazide-type diuretic — β-adrenergic blocking agent

FIGURE 6–5. The Step-Care method for the pharmacologic management of hypertension.

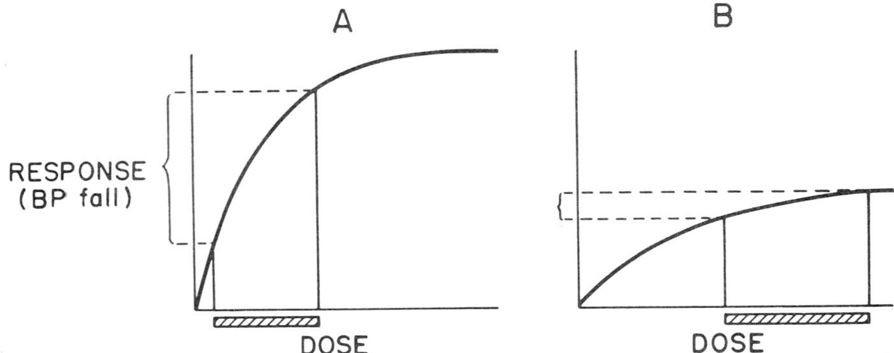

FIGURE 6–6. The two prototypical dose-response curves observed with antihypertensive agents. *A* represents a high dose-response relationship as might be obtained with guanethidine. Thus, up to a point, the more drug given, the greater the effect, and considerable care therefore is needed in regulating the dose. Conversely, *B* depicts a flat dose-response curve, as seen with thiazide diuretics and reserpine. With such drugs, once a certain dosage is reached, little if any further benefit is seen with larger doses. (Reproduced with permission from Kaplan, NM: Clinical Hypertension, 3rd ed. The Williams & Wilkins Co., Baltimore, 1982.)

In the next section, we will briefly review the rather basic pharmacology of a number of commonly used antihypertensive drugs. Following this survey, the selection of specific drugs for various types of hypertensive patients will be considered. The use of specific drugs in some of the secondary forms of hypertension (i.e., spironolactone in primary aldosteronism) will be considered subsequently in the respective chapters on the secondary hypertensive states.

Before we consider specific antihypertensive agents, a general point should be made about dose-response curves. As shown in Figure 6–6A, a progressively increased effect occurs throughout the therapeutic range. Thus, up to a point, the more drug given, the greater the effect, and considerable care therefore is needed in regulating the dose. This steep dose-response curve characterizes guanethidine and to a somewhat lesser degree, methyldopa, hydralazine, and propranolol. Conversely, Figure 6–6B depicts a flat dose-response curve, as seen with thiazide diuretics and reserpine. With such drugs, once a certain dosage is reached, little if any further benefit is seen with larger doses. Table 6–1 summarizes the mode of administration, major action, and important adverse effects of the commonly used antihypertensive agents.

DIURETICS

As noted earlier, despite a recent trend to use beta-adrenoceptor inhibitors as Step-1 drugs, diuretics still constitute the most commonly prescribed Step-1 medication in the United States. In the following section, we will briefly consider the attributes of several frequently used diuretic agents. For convenience, we will group these drugs into three classes:

1. Thiazide-like diuretics
2. Potassium-sparing diuretics

3. Diuretics with a major site of action in the loop of Henle—including furosemide, ethacrynic acid, and the recently released drug bumetanide.

Thiazide and Thiazide-like Diuretics

Chlorothiazide, chlorthalidone, and many other derivatives have been among the most widely used oral diuretics for treatment of hypertension. The various compounds differ primarily in dosage required and duration of action. Claims that they differ in a major way in their relative abilities to promote potassium excretion are probably unwarranted.

These diuretics act by inhibiting sodium and chloride reabsorption in the cortical diluting segment of the ascending limb of the loop of Henle. Plasma and extracellular fluid (ECF) volume are thereby diminished, and cardiac output falls. With chronic use, plasma volume and cardiac output returns partially toward normal, but at the same time peripheral resistance decreases. The decrease in peripheral resistance may involve a decrease in vascular reactivity to pressor stimuli. Although it has been postulated that such decreased vascular reactivity might reflect a reduction in sodium and water within the vessel walls, this could not be demonstrated in animals given thiazides chronically.

When used alone, thiazides produce a decrement in blood pressure after three to four weeks that varies from about 10/5 to 20/10 mm Hg. About 45 per cent of patients with mild hypertension can be expected to normalize their pressure with a thiazide alone.

Diuretics That Limit Potassium Losses

Three types of diuretics simultaneously promote sodium excretion and minimize potassium excretion (Table 6–2). All three influence transport processes primarily in the distal nephron. Such diuretics may be considered in patients requiring potassium repletion who do not comply with a regimen of potassium salts.

Spironolactone. Aldosterone promotes reabsorption of small amounts of sodium and accelerates distal tubular potassium and hydrogen ion secretion (and excretion). Spironolactone is a true competitive inhibitor of aldosterone at its renal site of action. Although the peak natriuretic effect of spironolactone administration is modest (excretion of less than 2 per cent of the filtered sodium chloride load), the cumulative effect of chronic administration may be substantial.

Triamterene. Triamterene, a pteridine derivative, has a direct effect on the distal tubule that results in both the inhibition of sodium chloride reabsorption and the retardation of potassium and hydrogen ion excretion. Thus, its antagonism of the renal tubular effects of aldosterone is indirect, and it is potassium-sparing even in patients with low or absent aldosterone levels (i.e., adrenalectomized subjects). This drug may also depress the glomerular filtration rate and renal blood flow. Like spironolactone, it interferes slightly with the excretion of water.

Amiloride. Amiloride is the most recently introduced potassium-sparing diuretic in the United States. Like triamterene, it impairs the reabsorption of sodium and the secretion of potassium in the distal nephron, independent of the level of circulating aldosterone. It has the potential, as do other potassium-sparing diuretics, to produce hyperkalemia and hyperchloremic metabolic acidosis. One advantage is its long duration of action, which permits a once-a-day dosage.

TABLE 6-1. COMMONLY USED ANTIHYPERTENSIVE MEDICATIONS

Specific Agents	Usual Dosage (in mg/day)	Major Action	Most Common or Important Complications	Conditions Often Requiring Modification of Usage, or Contraindications
DIURETICS				
Thiazides	Equivalent to hydrochlorothiazide, 25–100	Extracellular fluid (ECF) volume depletion	Hypokalemia, hyperuricemia, weakness and lassitude	Gout, simultaneous digitalization, renal failure, diabetes
Chlorthalidone	25–50	ECF volume contraction	As above	As above
Metolazone	2.5–5.0	ECF depletion; effective in renal failure	As above	As above
Indapamide	2.5–5.0	ECF volume contraction	As above	As above
Loop Diuretics				
Furosemide	40–80	As above	As above, plus dehydration and 8th nerve damage; with bumetanide, risk of ototoxicity uncertain	As above
Ethacrynic acid	50–100			
Bumetanide	0.5–2.0			
K-sparing Agents				
Spironolactone	25–100	Mild ECF contraction without hypokalemia. Serves as adjunct to thiazide-like or loop-active diuretic by limiting urinary potassium losses	Hyperkalemia, hyperchloremic acidosis, gynecomastia, irregular menses	Hyperkalemia, renal failure, diabetes
Triamterene	50–200	As above	Hyperkalemia, hyperchloremic acidosis, diarrhea, nausea	As above
Amiloride	5–10	As above	Hyperkalemia, hyperchloremic acidosis	As above

ADRENERGIC INHIBITORS

Noncardioselective Beta-Adrenoceptor Blockers				
Propranolol	80–320	Decreased cardiac output; decreased renin, central effect; blockade of prejunctional beta receptor	Bronchospasm, masking of hypoglycemia, angina or myocardial infarction after sudden drug withdrawal, pressor reactions during hypoglycemia, increased arteriolar constriction in vasospastic disorders	Heart block (greater than first degree), asthma, brittle insulin-dependent diabetes, overt congestive heart failure
Timolol	20–60	As above	As above	As above
Nadolol (long-acting)	80–320	As above	As above	As above
Cardioselective Beta-Adrenoceptor Blockers				
Metoprolol	100–400	As above	As above	As above
Atenolol (long-acting)	50–100	As above	As above	As above
ISA-positive Beta-Adrenoceptor Blockers				
Pindolol	15–45	As above	As above	As above
Oxprenolol	80–320	As above	As above	As above
Other Adrenergic Inhibitors				
Methyldopa	500–1000	Central autonomic inhibition	Weakness, lassitude, nightmares, Coombs-positive hemolytic anemia	Depression, liver disease
Clonidine	0.2–1.6	As above	Dry mouth, drowsiness or sedation, dizziness, discontinuation syndrome	Poor compliance
Guanabenz	8–32	As above	As above	As above
Prazosin	2–15	Inhibition of postsynaptic alpha-adrenergic receptor	Sodium retention, hypotension (esp. on initiation of therapy)	

Table continued on following page

TABLE 6–1.　COMMONLY USED ANTIHYPERTENSIVE MEDICATIONS *(Continued)*

Specific Agents	Usual Dosage (in mg/day)	Major Action	Most Common or Important Complications	Conditions Often Requiring Modification of Usage, or Contraindications
Reserpine	0.1–0.25	Central catecholamine depletion	Depression, peptic ulcer, decreased libido, nasal congestion	Peptic ulcer disease, psychiatric depression
Guanethidine	25 to 50 (start with 10 mg/day)	Postganglionic sympathetic blockade	Orthostatic and exercise hypotension, bradycardia, sexual dysfunction, diarrhea, edema	Known or suspected pheochromocytoma, frank congestive heart failure not due to hypertension, severe coronary artery or cerebrovascular disease
VASODILATORS				
Hydralazine	50–200	Decreased arteriolar resistance	Tachycardia, angina, headache, lupus-like reaction, sodium retention	Tachyarrhythmias, lupus erythematosus
Minoxidil	5–30	As above	Tachycardia, angina, hypertrichosis, edema, pericardial effusion	
ANGIOTENSIN-CONVERTING ENZYME INHIBITORS				
Captopril	37.5–150	Decrease of angiotensin II	Rash, loss of taste, hypotension, leukopenia, proteinuria	Serious impairment of renal function, serious autoimmune disease (particularly SLE), or exposure to other drugs known to affect white blood cells or immune response
CALCIUM-ENTRY BLOCKERS				
Nifedipine	20–40	Vasodilation by inhibition of influx of calcium into vascular	Hypotension, dizziness, flushing, tachycardia, periph-	Currently awaiting FDA approval as a medication for hy-

TABLE 6–2. POTENTIAL METABOLIC SIDE EFFECTS OF DIURETICS

Hypokalemia	Hyperuricemia
Metabolic alkalosis	Lipid abnormalities
Hyponatremia	Aggravation of carbohydrate intolerance
Hypercalcemia	Azotemia
Magnesium depletion	

Diuretics That Inhibit Sodium Chloride Transport in the Ascending Limb of Henle's Loop

Ethacrynic acid and furosemide are two potent loop-type diuretics that may be administered intravenously or by mouth. Furosemide may also be given intramuscularly. They are distinguished by their remarkable natriuretic activity (the amount of the filtered sodium chloride load that may be delivered into the urine may be several times greater than that accompanying the use of thiazide-type diuretics) and by the fact that their major site of action is in the thick ascending limb of Henle's loop. Although very dissimilar chemically, both ethacrynic acid and furosemide have many similar pharmacologic properties.

Bumetanide is a newly released loop-diuretic. Like furosemide it is a sulfonamide derivative with its major site of action in the ascending limb of the loop of Henle. It has a rapid onset and short duration of action. Whether bumetanide or the similar investigational agent piretanide has any advantages over the currently available loop diuretics remains to be determined.

Because of their great potency, the loop diuretics have a much greater propensity than thiazide-like agents for inducing fluid-electrolyte and acid-base abnormalities, some of which are severe.

Metabolic Fluid and Electrolyte Abnormalities Associated with Diuretic Therapy

Oral thiazide diuretics remain the most widely used treatment for hypertension. Many patients continue on therapy all their lives; the long-term metabolic consequences of thiazide diuretics are therefore of considerable importance. There are diverse potential metabolic fluid and electrolyte abnormalities associated with diuretic administration in the hypertensive patient (Table 6–2). Abnormalities indicated by metabolic variables such as serum potassium, glucose, cholesterol, and uric acid must be weighed against the benefits of treatment, which may be modest in patients with mild hypertension. Additional derangements include alkalosis, azotemia, and hyponatremia.

Table 6–3 shows the frequency of biochemical abnormalities resulting from

TABLE 6–3. PER CENT INCIDENCE OF BIOCHEMICAL ABNORMALITIES AFTER ONE YEAR OF TREATMENT WITH THIAZIDE DIURETICS

	Per Cent Incidence at One Year		
Blood Chemistry	PLACEBO CONTROL	DIURETIC-TREATED	INCREASED INCIDENCE IN TREATED GROUP
Uric acid > 7.9 mg/dl	16%	30%	14%
Potassium < 3.5 mEq/L	2%	23%	21%
Fasting glucose ≥ 110 mg/dl	16%	21%	5%

Data taken from Report of Veterans Administration Cooperative Study: Circulation 45:991–1004, 1972.

Reproduced with permission From Gifford, RW, Jr.: Hypertension Update 4:193, 1982.

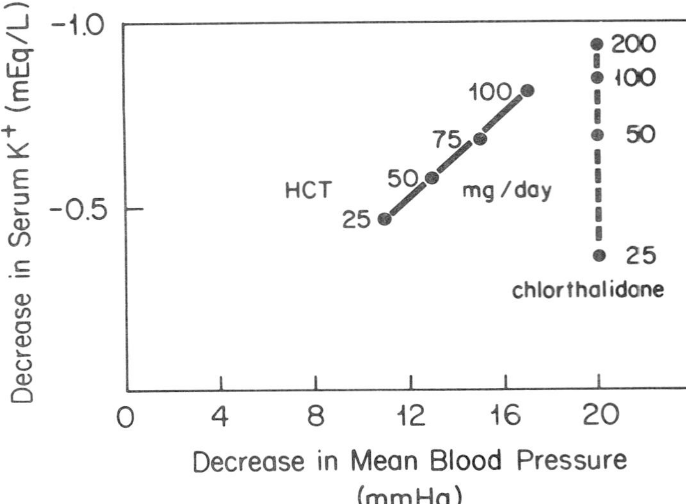

FIGURE 6–7. The effects of varying doses of hydrochlorothiazide and chlorthalidone on serum potassium and blood pressure of hypertensive patients. Increasing the dose of chlorthalidone does not further lower blood pressure but increases the risk of significant hypokalemia in an unacceptably high proportion of patients. Incremental doses of hydrochlorothiazide result in only a further modest lowering of blood pressure. (Reproduced with permission from Kaplan, NM: Clinical Hypertension, 3rd ed. The Williams & Wilkins Co., Baltimore, 1982.)

one year's treatment with thiazide-type diuretics. As is well known, these agents cause an increased incidence of hypokalemia, hyperuricemia, and hyperglycemia. A point to be noted, however, is that untreated hypertensive patients (placebo group) manifest a high incidence of hyperuricemia and hyperglycemia. Conversely, unprovoked hypokalemia is rare; thus, as already emphasized, its presence should raise the suspicion of a previously unrecognized case of primary aldosteronism.

Hypokalemia

Serum potassium levels fall below 3.5 mEq/L in approximately 10 per cent of patients with essential hypertension receiving thiazides chronically. Although it has been estimated that such patients incur potassium deficits averaging 200 mEq or less, the methodology for determining such losses is not rigorous. In fact, it has been proposed that the hypokalemia may be attributable in part to a translocation of potassium into cells without a net loss of the cation from the body. The variability in decrements in serum potassium levels and potassium depletion relates to several factors, including the dosage of diuretic, level of plasma aldosterone, acid-base status, pre-existing potassium balance, and sodium intake.

Figure 6–7 depicts the effects of varying doses of hydrochlorothiazide and chlorthalidone on serum potassium and blood pressure in two groups of hypertensive patients. Increasing the dose of chlorthalidone does not further lower blood pressure, but it does increase the risk of significant hypokalemia in an unacceptably high proportion of patients.

The dose-related increase in the frequency of biochemical side effects without an important corresponding augmentation of antihypertensive effect warrants the recommendation (recently reinforced by the World Health Organization) to prescribe diuretics only in relatively low doses.

What Should Alert the Physician to Hypokalemia: Clinical Symptoms, a Laboratory Determination, or Both? Clinically important hypokalemia may give rise to signs and symptoms that alert the physician to this abnormality. Some patients manifest symptoms such as fatigue, muscle cramps (usually in the lower extremities), and constipation. Occasionally, these symptoms may occur at serum potassium levels not usually considered particularly low (i.e., 3.2 to 3.4 mEq/L). Many hypokalemic patients, however, remain asymptomatic.

In view of the dissociation between symptoms and plasma potassium levels, how should we monitor this abnormality? Although the electrocardiogram may reflect alterations in potassium balance and serum potassium concentration, it is generally relatively insensitive for this purpose. Rather, the only practical approach to detecting hypokalemia is to monitor serum potassium levels periodically.

Should the Physician Routinely Administer Potassium Supplements to Hypertensive Patients Being Treated with Diuretics? It is clear that (in the absence of renal failure) potassium should be prescribed for hypertensive patients receiving concomitant digitalis medications and patients manifesting signs and symptoms referable to potassium depletion. Nevertheless, significant controversy attends the question whether there is a value in preventing potassium depletion in hypertensive patients receiving diuretics. *Should all hypertensive patients with diuretic treatment be placed on potassium supplements?*

More than five years ago, in a critical review, Kassirer and Harrington surveyed the available data and concluded that prophylactic potassium therapy should be restricted to a small subgroup. Their findings were as follows:

1. Hypertensive patients receiving thiazide diuretics alone or furosemide alone usually have a minimal or negligible degree of potassium deficiency.

2. Except in patients also receiving digitalis, no adverse consequences could be attributed to deficits of this magnitude.

3. A minority of diuretic-treated patients remain hypokalemic despite such prophylactic potassium supplementation.

4. Hyperkalemia constitutes a significant risk of treatment with potassium salts and potassium-sparing diuretics, particularly in diabetic patients, the elderly, and patients with impaired renal function. In one large series, the frequency of dangerous complications of oral potassium therapy was approximately one in 200.

From these observations, Kassirer and Harrington concluded that patients receiving diuretics should not routinely receive prophylactic treatment, but that periodic monitoring of serum potassium concentration is an appropriate precaution. Edematous, salt-restricted patients in whom alkalosis is likely to develop and patients receiving both digitalis and diuretics were excluded from these recommendations; in such patients deficiencies of both potassium and chloride should be avoided assiduously.

Despite scholarly reviews such as the one by Kassirer and Harrington, guidelines for potassium repletion in hypokalemic patients who do not take digitalis remained controversial, and very few data have become available about this widespread clinical problem. Some clinicians claim that patients tolerate hypokalemia quite well and recommend potassium repletion only when potassium depletion is more marked (serum K less than 3.0 mEq/L) or when the patient becomes symptomatic. In contrast, however, other clinicians have been concerned about certain recently recognized cardiovascular complications of diuretic-induced hypokalemia, particularly ventricular arrhythmias. Unfortunately, the incidence of ventricular ectopic activity in nondigitalized, hypokalemic patients remains unknown. The incidence of ventricular ectopic activity noted in retrospective studies with the routine electrocardiogram in nondigitalized patients has varied from eight per cent to 28 per cent. Such data are confounded by the realization that the routine electrocardiogram has very low sensitivity in identifying ventricular ectopic activity in comparison to other techniques, such as 24-hour ambulatory electrocardiographic monitoring and exercise testing.

In a recent study, Holland et al. prospectively assessed the incidence and types of ventricular ectopic activity during diuretic-induced hypokalemia in patients with essential hypertension and attempted to document the effect of potassium repletion. Patients without evidence of cardiac disease other than uncomplicated left ventricular hypertrophy were selected so that production of potassium depletion would pose less danger to the patient. They observed that ventricular ectopic activity developed in seven of 21 patients (33 per cent) during diuretic-induced hypokalemia. Nevertheless, they were unable to demonstrate that hypokalemia increases patient mortality or morbidity, since none of their patients died, and evidence of patient morbidity was minimal (palpitations in two patients noted only after direct questioning).

In another provocative study of 151 patients, Solomon and Cole assessed the importance of diuretic-induced hypokalemia as a determinant of ventricular arrhythmias in patients with an acute myocardial infarction. Sixty-seven per cent of patients with a serum potassium of less than 3.1 mEq/L had serious ventricular arrhythmias, compared with 40 per cent of patients with a serum potassium between 3.1 and 3.5 mEq/L and 20 per cent of normokalemic patients. The authors concluded that hypokalemia is not only a common problem in patients with acute myocardial infarction but also a clinically significant factor in the development of life-threatening arrhythmias.

Despite such arguments, in their most recent reappraisal of the problem, Harrington et al. again concluded that prophylactic potassium therapy should be restricted to a small population. These investigators reassessed the available data through 1981, including studies that used 24-hour electrocardiographic monitoring, and concluded that one is apparently dealing with "competing risks"—the risk of fatal arrhythmias in patients deprived of potassium prophylaxis and of fatal hyperkalemia in patients receiving potassium salts or potassium-sparing diuretics.

RECOMMENDATIONS. Since it is not yet established whether the risk of hyperkalemia in treated patients balances the risk of hypokalemia in untreated patients, we recommend that potassium salts or potassium-sparing diuretics not be prescribed routinely for diuretic-treated hypertensive patients. Rather, they should be reserved for those patients who are also receiving digitalis, those with potassium depletion (serum potassium less than 3.2 mEq/L), or those with clinical manifestations that can be clearly attributed to potassium deficiency. Whether patients with resting electrocardiographic abnormalities should be treated remains unanswered at present. Our recommendation is that such patients be treated prophylactically pending resolution of this question.

Which Potassium Salts Should Be Used as a Supplement? When the decision to replete potassium is made, the question invariably arises as to which potassium salts should be used. There is a consensus that for diuretic-induced hypokalemia, potassium chloride is the appropriate supplement. Diuretic-induced hypokalemia is usually associated with metabolic alkalosis, which predisposes the patient to further potassium loss. Thus, the expeditious correction of the concomitant alkalosis with chloride constitutes part of the therapeutic approach for appropriate potassium repletion. Whether one uses liquids, effervescent powders or granules, or slow-release tablets, the major considerations are patient preference (convenience), simplicity, safety, and cost.

Liquid or Tablet Forms of Potassium Chloride? Although liquid supplements

TABLE 6–4. SLOW-RELEASE POTASSIUM PREPARATIONS

Preparation	Manufacturer	Potassium per Capsule or Tablet (mEq)	Cost of 40 mEq
Micro-K	A. H. Robins	8	$.52
Kaon-Cl	Adria	6.7	.63
Kaon-Cl-10	Adria	10	.47
Klotrix	Mead Johnson	10	.50
K-Tab	Abbott	10	.45
Slow-K	Ciba	8	.50

Reproduced with permission from the Medical Letter 24:72, Aug. 6, 1982.

are safer than tablets, many patients find the liquids unpalatable. The most widely prescribed products are slow-release tablets containing potassium chloride in a wax matrix (Table 6–4). Rarely, these tablets can cause gastrointestinal ulceration, bleeding, obstruction, and perforation when the intestinal mucosa is exposed to high local concentrations of potassium. Since elderly or immobile patients are likely to have delayed gastrointestinal transit time, it is not always possible to detect these predisposing conditions. Recently, a slow-release capsule (Micro-K) has been promoted with the claim that it minimizes the possibility of damage to the gastrointestinal mucosa. The theoretic advantages of this preparation are the dispersion of the polymer-coated KCl in the gastrointestinal tract and the slow release of potassium in solution, both intended to avoid high local concentrations of potassium that could damage the mucosa. Whether the theoretic advantages of this product are borne out must await controlled trials and additional clinical experience.

Dosage. The usual dosage for prevention of hypokalemia is about 20 to 40 mEq of potassium daily; for treatment of potassium depletion, dosage varies from 40 to 100 mEq/day.

Can Salt Substitutes Be Effectively Used as Potassium Supplements? A frequent question is whether the patient can utilize one of the KCl- containing salt substitutes as a potassium supplement? The answer is probably yes. If a patient can tolerate the taste of these preparations, he can replace potassium at a much lower cost than with the commercial potassium supplements. As an example, a teaspoon of salt substitute per day is equivalent to 40 mEq per day of potassium supplements, at a cost of pennies.

Carbohydrate Abnormalities

The diabetogenic effect of thiazides has been widely reported, and its importance disputed. There is little doubt that thiazides may worsen diabetes in patients with established diabetes, but their role in provoking glucose intolerance in previously glucose-tolerant subjects is controversial. Dollery's group recently reported a statistically significant alteration in glucose tolerance commencing after six years' treatment with diuretics. The changes were more pronounced in a subsequent evaluation after 14 years. Furthermore, by World Health Organization (WHO) criteria, whereas only three of 34 patients had glucose intolerance before treatment, after 14 years six patients were diabetic and seven additional subjects were glucose intolerant. Of interest, Berglund and Andersson found no difference in the induction of glucose intolerance between patients with hypertension treated with beta-blockers and those treated with diuretics.

Hyperuricemia

Elevated plasma uric acid levels are observed in as many as 30 per cent of untreated hypertensive patients; thiazide therapy doubles this incidence. Furthermore, thiazide drugs may precipitate acute gouty arthritis in susceptible patients.

Since a preponderance of hypertensive patients manifest elevated uric acid levels either spontaneously or in association with thiazide therapy, it would be impractical either to avoid prescription of such drugs in hypertensive patients or to initiate measures to lower uric acid in all hyperuricemic hypertensive patients. Of greater importance, there is no compelling evidence that treatment of asymptomatic hyperuricemia is of benefit. Furthermore, as with other modes of therapy, it carries potential risks. Given these considerations, our own recommendation is that therapy with allopurinol or probenecid be initiated only in those patients with a personal or family history of gout or in those with plasma uric acid levels exceeding 11 mg/dl.

Hyponatremia

Hyponatremia is a quite uncommon but potentially serious complication of diuretic administration. Although it may occur, of course, as a result of marked urinary sodium losses, the term *diuretic-induced hyponatremia* presently is usually used to refer to a syndrome characterized by moderate to severe hyponatremia in the absence of clinically apparent contraction of the extracellular fluid volume. In fact, in the classic paper of Fichman et al., neither sodium deficit nor water excess was observed; i.e., the hyponatremia must have resulted at least in part from a redistribution of sodium and water. Some, but not all, studies have shown that the development of potassium deficiency is a prerequisite, and the presence of mild metabolic alkalosis is typical. This condition tends to appear in patients ingesting a large amount of water. They do not develop hemodilution, however, until the ability of their kidneys to excrete water becomes impaired as a result of the administration of various diuretics that have their site of action in the distal nephron (diluting segments). Thus, at least for some patients developing diuretic-induced hyponatremia, both excessive fluid intake and the use of an agent that impairs renal diluting ability (and perhaps causes hypokalemia) are necessary.

How does the physician suspect the presence of diuretic-induced hyponatremia aside from periodic surveillance of plasma electrolytes? Of course, if the hyponatremia is mild, the condition may be asymptomatic. On the other hand, more marked hyponatremia may be associated with any of a spectrum of symptoms ranging from simple weakness, fatigue, or anorexia to altered mental status and generalized seizures.

Why this condition is uncommon is not known. The syndrome abates promptly upon discontinuation of the diuretic and sometimes can be prevented by KCl supplementation or restriction of water intake. Obviously, if withdrawal of the diuretic ameliorates, but does not completely correct, the hyponatremia, another etiology, such as syndrome of inappropriate antidiuretic hormone secretion (SIADH), must be looked for.

Metabolic Alkalosis

Both thiazide-type and loop-active diuretics commonly induce mild hypochloremic metabolic alkalosis, almost always in association with hypokalemia. In the patient with essential hypertension, this adverse effect appears to be of limited clinical importance. Nevertheless, the clinician should not be surprised at the finding of modestly elevated levels of serum [HCO_3] on routine laboratory surveillance.

A corollary of practical importance is that the presence of alkalosis influences the approach to the treatment of hypokalemia in the hypertensive patient. In this instance, the use of the chloride salt of potassium is preferable, both to permit potassium repletion and to correct the alkalosis.

Hypercalcemia

An increase in serum calcium is a well-recognized complication of thiazide therapy. Although thiazides diminish the renal excretion of calcium, the cause of this phenomenon remains unclear and may involve potentiation of the effect of parathyroid hormone on bone. In the patient without an underlying abnormality of calcium homeostasis, only rarely do serum calcium levels exceed 11.0 mg/dl. On the other hand, if latent hyperparathyroidism is present, frank and sometimes severe hypercalcemia may ensue. Accordingly, it seems reasonable to recommend that when a patient receiving thiazides develops clear-cut hypercalcemia, he should be evaluated for primary hyperparathyroidism or another disorder of calcium homeostasis.

Prerenal Azotemia

Volume depletion is a common complication of diuretic use. This complication is particularly likely to occur in patients who are unable to replace urinary losses because of nausea, or when nonurinary losses are excessive, as with vomiting and diarrhea. Volume depletion may result in a diminished GFR, a resultant increase in blood urea nitrogen (BUN), and prerenal azotemia.

The Rational Use of Diuretics

The following specific remarks should be considered in relation to the prescribing of thiazide-type diuretics. These medications are relatively easy to use, since dose titration is simple. For example, when employing hydrochlorothiazide, one starts with 25 mg twice a day and increases this to 50 mg twice daily if the desired response is not achieved. Increasing the total daily dose of these medications above what corresponds to 100 mg of hydrochlorothiazide does not generally provide a greater reduction of blood pressure and may increase the risk of undesirable side effects. It is better at this point to add a Step-2 medication.

On the other hand, particularly if a patient's untreated hypertension is mild, a lower than usual dose may be sufficient and will tend to produce fewer metabolic derangements. Using a smaller dose of diuretic initially may be especially wise in the treatment of elderly patients with mainly systolic hypertension (see Chapter 11).

In general, it makes sense to use a long-acting diuretic such as chlorthalidone or metolazone for the treatment of hypertension. This simplifies the therapeutic regimen and tends to protect against sodium retention during the part of the day in which a short-acting agent may no longer be effective.

An optimal blood pressure response to the administration of a thiazide-type diuretic is a reduction of approximately 10 to 15 mm Hg systolic and 5 to 10 mm Hg diastolic. On initial consideration, one might anticipate that, because of their greater natriuretic potency, the loop-acting diuretics would induce a greater reduction in blood pressure than thiazide-type agents. Nevertheless, it has been clearly established that loop-diuretics do not exert a greater antihypertensive effect. Indeed, the results of a few studies suggest that thiazides exert a greater blood pressure–lowering effect. There is a specific setting, however, in which loop-diuretics are preferred. When a reduction of GFR (estimated by creatinine clearance) to a level of less than approximately 25 to 35 ml/min (serum creatinine generally about 2 to 2.5 mg/dl) has occurred, the efficacy of thiazide-type medications tends to diminish, mandating the use of a loop-active agent.

There are very few contraindications to the use of diuretics for the treatment of hypertension, and most patients tolerate these drugs rather well. A history of prior allergic reaction to a diuretic (or pancreatitis) contraindicates its future use. One should keep in mind that, except for ethacrynic acid and spironolactone (a weak diuretic generally not used by itself to treat essential hypertension), all of the commonly used diuretics are sulfonamide derivatives. Thus, because of the sulphur moiety, patients may rarely prove allergic to several otherwise chemically distinct medications.

One of the common mistakes incurred in the management of hypertensive patients is the use of improper dosages of medication. It must be emphasized that smaller doses of diuretic than many physicians have been using will provide most, if not all, of the antihypertensive action that diuretics are capable of providing, while simultaneously diminishing the degree of hypokalemia. The trade-off between the antihypertensive effect and the degree of potassium loss is summarized in Figure 6–2. As can be seen, increasing the dose of chlorthalidone from 25 to 50 mg per day does not increase the antihypertensive effect, but it increases the magnitude of hypokalemia. Similarly, increasing the dose of hydrochlorothiazide from 25 to 50 mg per day, and ultimately to 100 mg per day, has minimal additional hypotensive effect but increases hypokalemia.

Dietary Sodium Restriction as an Adjunct to Diuretics

The question is often asked concerning the appropriate level of sodium intake for a patient taking diuretics to treat essential hypertension. Our suggestion is to recommend a moderate restriction of dietary sodium intake. On the other hand, excessive sodium intake not infrequently appears to obviate the negative sodium balance that is the major basis for diuretic-induced antihypertensive effects.

Although there are considerable geographic and cultural differences, the typical American diet contains approximately 150 to 200 mEq of sodium per day. The exclusion of highly salted foods and the avoidance of adding salt in the preparation of food or at the table can be expected to reduce sodium intake to the range of 75 to 100 mEq of sodium per day. The reduction of sodium intake to levels less than 75 mEq per day is accomplished only with great difficulty and with significant added expense. Furthermore, in the absence of imaginative food preparation such diets tend to be quite unpalatable.

Of interest, a recent carefully conducted study by Ram et al. has shown that moderate dietary sodium restriction (to a level of approximately 70 mEq per day) in conjunction with diuretic administration increases the antihypertensive response and attenuates diuretic-induced urinary potassium losses. Furthermore, it was suggested that this dietary regimen plus a single morning dose of a diuretic of intermediate duration of action, such as hydrochlorothiazide, offers the best balance of safety and efficacy.

Another advantage of moderate sodium restriction may be a decrease in the required dosage of the diuretic or other antihypertensive medication. Finally, as mentioned above, preliminary data suggest that ingestion of a diet having a relatively high potassium to sodium ratio may contribute (because of the high potassium content) to blood pressure reduction.

Potassium-sparing Diuretics

In addition to the controversy surrounding the potassium deficits induced by diuretics, the clinician may be confused by the deluge of promotional material suggesting that this problem can be obviated by prescribing potassium-sparing diuretics. The differential features of the three currently available potassium-sparing diuretics are given in Table 6–5.

Do these agents indeed provide a panacea? Our own impression is that the problem is not nearly so easily solved and that potassium-sparing diuretics should be prescribed with circumspection for the following reason: All three of the potassium-sparing agents have the potential to induce severe hyperkalemia in many clinical settings in which potassium metabolism is already somewhat impaired or threatened. These situations include the following:

1. Clinical Disorders
   a. Hyporeninemic hypoaldosteronism
   b. Decreased renal reserve (as in the elderly patient)

2. Concomitant use of other medications
   a. Beta-adrenergic blockers
   b. Nonsteroidal anti-inflammatory agents
   c. Captopril
   d. Potassium supplements

Normal potassium homeostasis requires sufficient renal function to permit appropriate potassium excretion. Both tubular function and GFR are important. Any drug or condition that alters renal function may impair the ability to excrete potassium.

Hyporeninemic Hypoaldosteronism. The syndrome of hyporeninemic hypoaldosteronism (SHH) is the most common form of isolated mineralocorticoid deficiency in the adult. Typically, it is observed in patients with mild to moderate renal insufficiency related either to some form of chronic interstitial nephritis or, more commonly, to diabetic nephropathy. Hyperkalemia and hyperchloremic metabolic acidosis are the characteristic laboratory abnormalities. The hyperkalemia appears to relate primarily to hypoaldosteronism in the setting of decreased GFR. Frequently, but not invariably, it responds to the administration of fludrocortisone, a potent mineralocorticoid. Not surprisingly, patients with SHH are at risk of exacerbation of their hyperkalemia by the administration of medications, such as potassium-sparing diuretics, that further perturb the external balance of potassium.

Decreased Renal Reserve in the Elderly. Renal function declines with advancing age, and normal subjects at the age of 80 may have glomerular filtration rates as low as 50 per cent of normal, i.e., in the range of about 50 ml/min. Since muscle mass (and creatinine production) generally decreases pari passu there is no increase in serum creatinine concentration. One must either measure creatinine clearance or use an age-weight serum creatinine formula such as that derived by Cockcroft and Gault to estimate GFR. Under ordinary circumstances, the decrement in renal function associated with aging is of limited clinical importance. Two examples, however, in which it may be of significance are in the increased risk of aminoglycoside-induced acute tubular necrosis and the increased potential for hyperkalemia upon administration of potassium supplements or potassium-sparing diuretics.

TABLE 6–5. FEATURES OF POTASSIUM-SPARING DIURETICS

Diuretic	Antagonism of Aldosterone, per se	Direct Tubular Effect	Potential for Production of Hyperkalemia	Production of Hyperchloremic Acidosis	Relative Contraindication		Long-Acting
					RENAL FAILURE	CONCOMITANT USE OF POTASSIUM SUPPLEMENTATION	
Spironolactone	+	−	+	+	+	+	−
Triamterene	−	+	+	+	+	+	−
Amiloride	−	+	+	+	+	+	+

Beta-Adrenergic Blockers. Certain patients receiving beta-adrenergic blocking drugs are at risk of developing hyperkalemia, if they have coexistent disorders affecting potassium homeostasis. At least two mechanisms contribute to the development of hyperkalemia: (a) suppression of aldosterone with a diminution of potassium excretion and (b) alteration of autonomic function with the resultant disturbance of internal potassium homeostasis.

Nonsteroidal Anti-inflammatory Drugs (NSAID). Patients receiving nonsteroidal anti-inflammatory drugs are at risk of developing hyperkalemia. Although the frequency with which this side effect occurs is not established, it may be catastrophic. There are several mechanisms whereby NSAID drugs may produce hyperkalemia. These include suppression of aldosterone, with a decrease in potassium excretion. Theoretically, the decrease in sodium delivery to the distal nephron believed to occur with NSAID administration may also favor an impairment of potassium excretion.

Conclusion

Given the above caveats, what is the role of the potassium-sparing diuretics in the management of patients with essential hypertension? In the prudent diuretic management of patients with one of the edematous states, such as cirrhosis of the liver, who are particularly prone to the development of hypokalemia and metabolic alkalosis, these agents may be of major importance. On the other hand, it is our opinion that their place in the treatment of essential hypertension is more secondary, and we reserve their use for those relatively exceptional individuals who develop symptomatic or worrisome hypokalemia and do not tolerate or are noncompliant with a regimen of potassium supplements. Finally it must be emphasized that the concomitant administration of potassium supplements together with potassium-sparing diuretics is contraindicated, with extremely rare exceptions.

ADRENERGIC INHIBITORS

Beta-Adrenoceptor Blockers

The prominence devoted in this chapter to beta-blockers will be immediately apparent to the reader. There are several reasons for this, including the growing importance of these agents as antihypertensive medications (40 per cent of the nondiuretic U.S. market in 1980 as opposed to only 13 per cent in 1978), the several medications in this class now available in the United States, the somewhat bewildering panoply of similar and distinguishing features of the individual agents, and the potentially beneficial and adverse aspects of their use in combination with other blood pressure–lowering medications.

Mechanism of Antihypertensive Action. In spite of many years of use and investigation, the mechanism(s) whereby beta-blockers lower blood pressure has not been fully elucidated. The fact that theories abound indicates the lack of consensus. Certainly the reduction of cardiac output, readjustment of peripheral resistance, and, in some instances, reduction of PRA play a role. A recent suggestion that may prove important is that beta-blockers inhibit prejunctional beta receptors. Figure 6–4 depicts in schematic fashion the peripheral sympathetic nerve terminal and illustrates how presynaptic beta-blockade might reduce vasoconstriction by leading to inhibition of norepinephrine release. Finally, it has been postulated that alterations of the prostaglandin and kinin system may be involved.

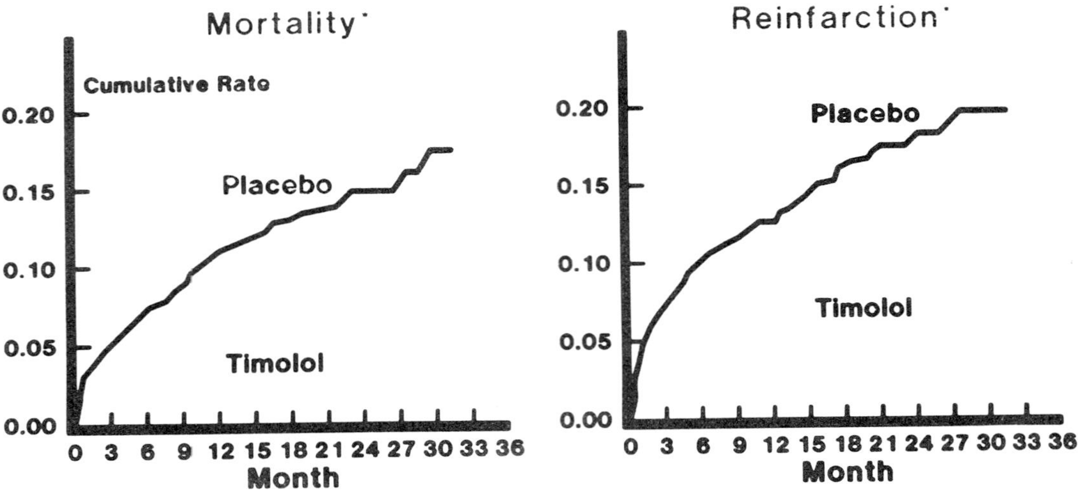

FIGURE 6–8. Cardioprotective effects of a beta-blocker in a study of 1884 patients. As can be seen, in comparison to placebo, timolol conferred protection against reinfarction and mortality in patients who had suffered a previous myocardial infarction. As noted in the text, this cardioprotective advantage has been observed with several of the beta-blockers. (Modified from the Norwegian Multicenter Study Group. Reprinted by permission of the New England Journal of Medicine 304:801–807, 1981.)

At the time of writing there are seven beta-blocking agents available in the United States for the treatment of hypertension. All beta-blocking agents share in common certain features, i.e., reduction in heart rate and a negative inotropic effect, reduction of blood pressure, reduction of the frequency of angina, and protection against sudden death and a second myocardial infarction (Fig. 6–8). Nevertheless, they differ in their secondary pharmacologic and physical properties (Table 6–6). These include intrinsic sympathomimetic activity (ISA), cardioselectivity or beta-1 selectivity, water versus lipid solubility, and membrane-stabilizing activity (MSA). The relevance of these properties to clinical usage will be considered in detail.

Table 6–7 summarizes the data regarding the major distinguishing features of the available beta-blockers. Although these pharmacologic differences have been well characterized, for the most part their established clinical importance is relatively limited. Exceptions, however, may be the relative cardioselectivity

TABLE 6–6. DISTINGUISHING PHYSICAL AND PHARMACOLOGIC FEATURES OF BETA-BLOCKERS

1. Cardioselectivity
2. Intrinsic sympathomimetic activity
3. Membrane-stabilizing activity
4. Solubility characteristics
    a. Hepatic first pass
    b. Reproducibility of blood level
    c. Duration of action
    d. Effect of renal failure
    e. Penetrability into central nervous system

TABLE 6–7. DIFFERENTIAL FEATURES OF BETA-ADRENOCEPTOR ANTAGONISTS

Agent	Cardio-selectivity	Intrinsic Sympathomimetic Activity	Membrane-stabilizing Activity	High Water Solubility
Propranolol (Inderal)	0	0	+	0
Metoprolol (Lopressor)	+	0	0	0
Nadolol (Corgard)	0	0	0	+
Atenolol (Tenormin)	+	0	0	+
Timolol (Blocadren)	0	0	0	0
Pindolol (Visken)	0	+	0	0
Oxprenolol (Trasicor)	0	+	+	0

of some agents, the intrinsic sympathomimetic activity of pindolol and oxprenolol, and the solubility characteristics of nadolol and atenolol.

The membrane-stabilizing activity (MSA) or quinidine-like action of propranolol does not actually obtain with clinically used dosages and is not relevant except perhaps in the case of a massive overdose or within the first few minutes of an intravenous dose.

Another feature is the solubility characteristics of these agents. Figure 6–9 depicts the relative water vs. lipid solubility of some of the available beta-blockers. As can be seen, propranolol is at the lipid solubility end of the continuum, whereas atenolol is the most water soluble of the agents. The relatively highly water-soluble agents are not appreciably metabolized in the liver, which probably accounts for their long duration of action, the greater predictability and reproducibility of the blood level following any given dosage, and the need to reduce the dosage in patients with renal failure to avoid the possibility of drug accumulation. In addition, the water-soluble medications appear to enter the central nervous system to a lesser degree. Although claims have been made that this property results in less fatigue, insomnia, nightmares, and depression, this has not been well established (Fig. 6–10).

Cardioselectivity. Various tissues and organs contain two distinct types of beta-receptors. Beta-1 receptors predominate in the heart, kidneys, and adipose tissue. Their stimulation increases heart rate, facilitates electrical conduction,

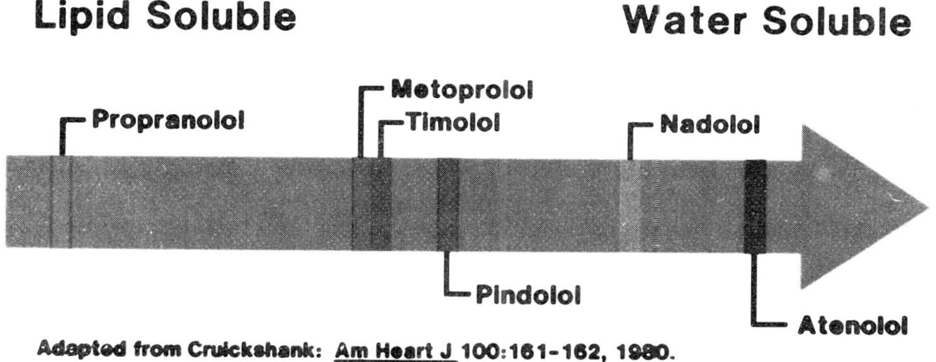

FIGURE 6–9. The relative water vs. lipid solubility of some of the available beta-blockers. As can be seen, propranolol is at the lipid solubility end of the continuum, whereas atenolol is the most soluble. (Adapted from Cruickshank: Am Heart J *100*:161–162, 1980.)

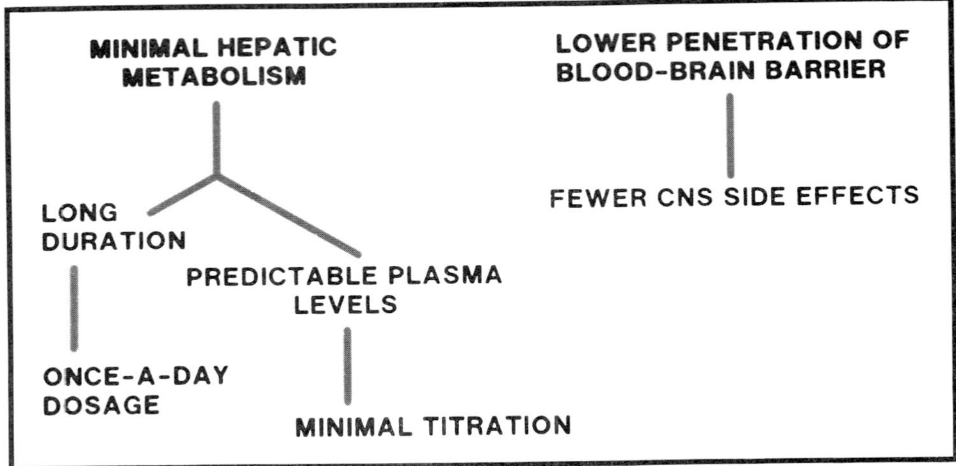

FIGURE 6–10. The potential advantage of water solubility. As can be seen, possibly as a consequence of a lower penetration of the blood-brain barrier, the incidence of central nervous system side effects appears to be lower. The advantage of reduced hepatic metabolism is a more predictable plasma level and a longer duration of action. Thus, dose titration is minimized, and dosage may be once a day. (Adapted from Cruickshank: Am Heart J *100*:161–162, 1980.)

enhances the force of myocardial contraction, augments the release of renin into the renal veins, and increases lipolysis. Blockade produces bradycardia, decreased cardiac output, eventual reduction in blood pressure, and inhibition of renin release. In contrast, beta-2 receptors predominate in the bronchi, arteriolar smooth muscle, and pancreas. Stimulation of these receptors causes bronchodilation, arteriolar dilation, insulin release, and lactate production, whereas inhibition is associated with the potential for bronchoconstriction, arteriolar constriction, and decreased insulin release and lactate formation. Figure 6–11 depicts in schematic fashion the relative distribution of beta-1 and beta-2 receptor sites. Beta-1 blockade generally produces the therapeutic features of adrenoceptor inhibition. Although blockade of the beta-2 receptor accounts for many of the undesirable side effects of beta-blockers, the frequency of other side effects is very much the same for all types of beta-blockers.

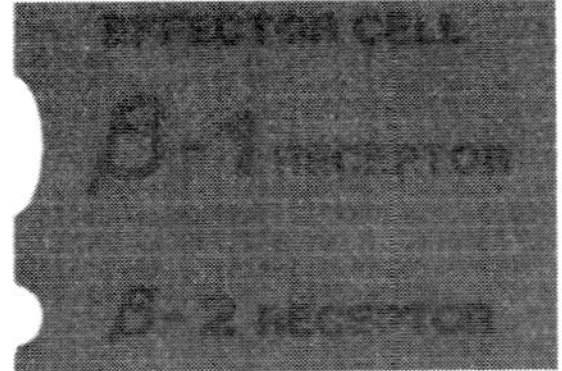

- **HEART**
- **KIDNEY RENIN RELEASE**

- **BRONCHI**
- **PERIPHERAL BLOOD VESSELS**
- **UTERUS**
- **INSULIN (PANCREAS)**
- **LACTIC ACID PRODUCTION**

FIGURE 6–11. A schematic depiction of the relative distribution of beta-1 and beta-2 receptor sites. As can be seen, although the indicated target sites contain both beta-1 and beta-2 receptors, the former predominate in the heart and kidney. Conversely, beta-2 receptors predominate in other target sites, including bronchi and peripheral blood vessels. (Adapted from Cruickshank: Am Heart J *100*:160, 1980.)

TABLE 6–8. POTENTIAL ADVANTAGES OF CARDIOSELECTIVE AGENTS

1. Allow wider patient selection
2. Possibly preferable to noncardioselective drugs in terms of the following:
    a. Bronchospasm
    b. Bronchodilator response to sympathomimetic agents
    c. Peripheral blood flow
    d. Peripheral resistance
    e. Diabetic patients

Cardioselectivity refers to the property of such agents as metoprolol and atenolol to inhibit beta-1 receptors to a greater extent than beta-2 receptors. It should be emphasized that cardioselectivity is a relative rather than an absolute feature. It tends to diminish as the dosage of medication increases into the range necessary for the management of many patients with moderate to severe hypertension. Cardioselectivity is important, but not in terms of efficacy of blood pressure lowering. Although, theoretically, stress- or exercise-induced increases in blood pressure would tend to be prevented by selective as opposed to nonselective agents, as already mentioned, all beta-blockers appear to have a similar ability to correct hypertension. What selectivity does confer is the advantage of a somewhat lesser risk of bronchospasm, vasospasm, and interference with carbohydrate metabolism in the predisposed patient who is considered to require the use of beta-adrenoceptor inhibition (Table 6–8).

ISA. Intrinsic sympathomimetic activity or partial agonistic activity (PAA) refers to the property of simultaneously blocking a beta-adrenoceptor yet acting to stimulate partially either the same or other beta receptors. This property is identified by slight cardiac stimulation that can be blocked by propranolol. Although the clinical importance of this pharmacologic feature requires further study and elucidation, there are theoretic considerations indicating that such an attribute may reduce the risk of some of the unwanted physiologic consequences of beta-blockade. In addition, there is preliminary clinical evidence suggesting that ISA-positive agents actually do have advantages over other agents not possessing this feature. As shown in Table 6–9, ISA tends to limit adverse effects on a number of target organs, including the heart, the lung, and the peripheral vasculature.

With regard to the heart, ISA-positive agents produce less bradycardia and do not reduce the cardiac output in the resting state. Furthermore, recent studies have demonstrated that in the patient with ischemic heart disease, the detrimental influence on left ventricular function during exercise is much less (less increase of pulmonary artery wedge pressure). Moreover, a physiologic

TABLE 6–9. POTENTIAL ADVANTAGES OF ISA-POSITIVE AGENTS

1. Allow broader patient selection
2. Possibly preferable to propranolol in terms of the following:
    a. Less bradycardia
    b. Less risk of congestive heart failure
    c. No increase in peripheral resistance
    d. Less worsening of peripheral vascular disease
    e. Less bronchospasm
    f. Less risk of withdrawal syndrome

variable that encompasses numerous factors, exercise tolerance, appears to be less impaired with ISA-positive agents. Thus, it appears that, in general, ISA-positive medications, as opposed to those agents lacking in this property, tend to support the mechanical and electrical activity of the heart.

With regard to pulmonary function, some but not all studies have shown that ISA-positive drugs induce a lessened decrease in mean expiratory flow rate.

An important attribute of ISA-positive beta-blockers is that they do not cause increases in total peripheral resistance. In fact, they tend to decrease peripheral resistance below the elevated pretreatment level, which is the prototypical hemodynamic abnormality of essential hypertension. As a result of this feature, signs and symptoms referable to decreased peripheral blood flow appear to be less common. For example, a side effect induced by beta-blockers that is seen with less frequency with ISA-positive drugs is a decrease in finger temperature. The latter is discernible by the patient as a very unpleasant symptom. Similarly, paresthesias also occur less frequently with ISA-positive drugs than with beta-blockers lacking in ISA.

Finally, withdrawal symptoms sometimes observed in patients who abruptly discontinue beta-blockers appear to be less prevalent with ISA-positive beta-blocking agents; perhaps because the up-regulation of receptor density (the increase in the number of beta receptors per unit area of target tissue that attends chronic beta-blocker administration) is diminished with the use of agents having partial agonist activity.

Contraindications. Beta-blockers are contraindicated in patients with frank congestive heart failure, asthma, greater than first-degree heart block, and severe peripheral vascular disease. They should be used with caution in patients concurrently receiving catecholamine-depleting drugs, such as reserpine, or medications containing sympathomimetic components, such as nasal decongestant sprays or drops (see Table 7–1).

Side Effects. When beta-blockers are appropriately withheld from use in patients, such as asthmatics, in whom their administration is contraindicated, adverse effects are infrequent, usually short-lived, and mild. The most common side effects include cold extremities, tiredness, lightheadedness, abdominal cramps, diarrhea or constipation, and insomnia. Exercise intolerance (particularly in athletic individuals), sexual dysfunction, and depression are sometimes noted. Bronchospasm and congestive heart failure are only rarely observed in patients without prior history of these conditions, but are not infrequently exacerbated when they have occurred previously. Recently, it has been observed that not only diuretics but also beta-blockers tend to impair lipid metabolism in that they increase plasma triglycerides and decrease plasma HDL–cholesterol concentration. It appears that nonselective beta-blockers without ISA do this to a greater extent than nonselective beta-blockers with ISA, while in relation to these two groups, the selective beta-blockers have an intermediate effect. Although collectively, the changes are in a direction that might exert deleterious effects with regard to the risk of coronary heart disease, there is no evidence at this time establishing such a risk.

Congestive Heart Failure. A frequently asked question is whether beta-blockers can be used safely in patients who have cardiomegaly (as assessed by chest x-ray) in the absence of overt congestive heart failure. Generally, the administration of beta-blockers in this setting is safe. Indeed, it has been proposed that such treatment may improve cardiac performance by reducing the elevated afterload characteristic of hypertension. Prudence dictates, however, that such patients be examined and questioned on each visit for evidence of signs or symptoms of cardiac decompensation.

Another often-asked question is whether the risk of side effects with beta-blockers increases coterminously with increasing dosage. The side effects that are most important in terms of potential severity relate to beta-blockade, and there is no clear-cut relationship between dose and the risk of side effects. For example, the patient who develops overt congestive heart failure, severe bradycardia, or bronchospasm usually manifests these complications at the doses typically employed to initiate antihypertensive therapy. Contrariwise, the patient who has not developed such serious adverse effects at low or moderate doses of beta-blockers is quite unlikely to manifest them at higher dose levels. This point is worth underscoring, because clinicians often inappropriately fail to increase the dose of beta-blockers for fear of side effects.

Beta-Blockers and Renal Function. Since long-standing, poorly controlled hypertension is an important cause of chronic renal failure, and therapy of hypertension may result at least temporarily in decrements in renal function, one of the sought-after attributes of antihypertensive agents has been the relative preservation of renal function. Recently, several studies have somewhat surprisingly revealed that some beta-blockers may adversely affect renal function. We have recently reviewed this topic in detail. In brief, the chronic use of propranolol is characterized by decrements of renal plasma flow and GFR of 10 to 20 per cent. The effect appears to persist for the duration of therapy and sometimes is progressive. In contrast, the long-term use of nadolol, probably atenolol, and perhaps other cardioselective agents appears to be relatively unassociated with impaired renal function. The mechanism of nephrotoxicity is probably hemodynamic and related to both diminished cardiac output and increased renal vascular resistance. The predisposing factors are uncertain. The clinical importance of these observations is presently unknown and is probably insignificant in patients whose underlying renal function is normal. We suggest that if renal function declines during chronic therapy with propranolol, one should consider switching to nadolol or atenolol (in a dose appropriate to the level of renal function) or to an antihypertensive agent of a different class, such as clonidine, methyldopa, or prazosin.

Discontinuation Syndrome. As is the case with other antihypertensives (see Chapter 9), beta-adrenoceptor inhibitors have also been inculpated with regard to the discontinuation syndrome. Abrupt termination of therapy with several beta-blockers has been reported to be associated with severe withdrawal symptoms. These include various signs of sympathetic overactivity, unmasking of hyperthyroidism, tachyarrhythmias, sudden death, aggravation of angina in patients with underlying coronary artery disease, and acute myocardial infarction. Symptoms of ischemic heart disease appear to occur mainly in a limited number of predisposed cardiac patients who have been given beta-blockers to treat angina as opposed to using them for hypertension alone. As mentioned above, the risk of this problem does not appear to be the same for the various agents. In particular, the ISA-positive drugs seem to have a reduced propensity to be associated with withdrawal symptoms. Withdrawal symptoms usually abate with reinstitution of beta-blocker therapy and can be prevented by gradual tapering of dosage over several days, particularly when the dosage has been high. Appropriate limitation of strenuous activity during withdrawal has also been recommended. Since patients with chronic hypertension probably have a high incidence of latent coronary artery disease, it is best to taper beta-adrenergic inhibitors in all patients, not just those with overt ischemic heart disease.

Clinical Usage and Dosage. Beta-blocking agents have become increasingly popular as Step-2 drugs because of their efficacy and relative lack of side effects compared with other sympatholytic agents. Recently, beta-blockers have also been widely used as the initial antihypertensive drug. This trend began mainly in Europe and has gained momentum elsewhere, including the United States, partly as a result of studies indicating that beta-blockers may be equally effective in lowering blood pressure but lacking some of the adverse metabolic side effects that attend diuretic administration. (For an in-depth discussion of the relative merits of diuretics vs. beta-blockers as the initial antihypertensive drug, see Chapter 8.)

When beta-blockers are administered orally their antihypertensive onset of action is approximately 24 hours. The maximal antihypertensive effect of any given dose is generally observed within one to two weeks. Therefore, if the antihypertensive response is inadequate after two weeks, the dose should be increased.

Since the various agents have a similar spectrum of therapeutic cardiovascular effects, if one agent in an appropriate dose does not lower blood pressure effectively, neither will another. Likewise, it is not helpful to add one beta-blocker to a second.

With beta-blockers, as with other inhibitors of components of the sympathetic nervous system, there is an increasing blood pressure–lowering effect when the dosage is changed from the initial low dosage levels to moderate dosage levels. Subsequently, however, further increasing the dose results in a relatively limited additional antihypertensive effect. Thus, the dose-response curve for beta-blockers is relatively flat, although not so flat as that seen with diuretic agents. For example, when doses of propranolol reach a level of approximately 240 mg/day, much of the potential antihypertensive effect has already been attained. Atenolol is the simplest of the beta-blockers to titrate, since it is recommended to begin with a daily dose of 50 mg, with one increment to twice this amount if an insufficient response is produced.

In general, the dosage range varies from one beta-blocker to another, and limitations of space prevent a full discussion herein (see Table 6–1). With propranolol, we recommend an initial dose for hypertension of 40 mg twice daily. In outpatients this can be gradually increased to a maximum of about 360 to 480 mg per day. Although preliminary evidence suggests that in sufficient dosage many of the relatively short-acting beta-blockers, such as propranolol and metoprolol, may be used once daily with satisfactory results, we presently limit such usage to the longer-acting products, atenolol and nadolol.

An interesting and recently recognized property of the beta-blockers is their ability to moderate the rise in both heart rate and systolic blood pressure during exercise (in contrast to the lack of modulation during methyldopa and clonidine therapy). Since the goal of treatment is to control blood pressure not only during sedentary activity but throughout the day, this property of beta-blockers may be of clinical importance in the selection of an antihypertensive drug.

Beta-Blockers in the Elderly. Are beta-blockers appropriate antihypertensive agents in the elderly? Although the available evidence suggests that beta-blockers may be less efficacious in older patients, perhaps because the elderly tend to have lower PRA levels, recent information indicates that this generalization may not always obtain.

Selection of a Beta-Blocking Agent. How should the clinician cope with the deluge of promotional material, which is appearing at an ever escalating rate, regarding the various beta-adrenoceptor blocking agents? Are the differences that are so heavily touted by the manufacturers of major importance? It appears that for the overwhelming majority of patients, since the anti-hypertensive efficacy of the beta-blockers is similar, other considerations are of relatively limited importance. Thus, in the majority of patients the choice of the beta-blocker should be based on the usual considerations of cost, frequency of administration, and the side effect profile. In the remaining minority of patients (estimated to constitute approximately 20 per cent of patients), differences encompassing cardioselectivity, presence of ISA, and other such factors may dictate the choice of the beta-blocking agent. Even in such patients, however, one has to remember that cardioselectivity is relative and dose related, and the principal effect of ISA-positive medications remains beta-blockade. Thus, all beta-blockers, including cardioselective and ISA-positive agents, are contraindicated in asthmatics. Similarly, although ISA-positive agents appear to be less likely to worsen peripheral vascular disease or congestive heart failure, patients with these conditions should be closely followed when treated with any beta-blocker.

In light of the advent of new beta-blocking agents with advantageous features, including water solubility, cardioselectivity, and the presence of ISA, it appears that the role of propranolol, the time-honored beta-adrenoceptor blocking agent in the treatment of hypertension, may have been supplanted.

The optimal regimen for the gradual withdrawal of beta-adrenoceptor inhibitors remains controversial. At this time we advise a slow tapering over a period of approximately two weeks, particularly if high doses have been used. The patient should be advised to avoid strenuous exercise during the withdrawal period and to report any adverse effects promptly.

Reserpine

Reserpine is one of several alkaloids of the Indian snakeroot plant. It acts by blocking the transport of norepinephrine into its storage granules, so that less of the neurotransmitter is available when the adrenergic nerves are stimulated. Consequently, sympathetic tone decreases, with a resultant decrease in peripheral vascular resistance. The effects are cumulative over at least two weeks.

Although reserpine has a relatively limited antihypertensive effect by itself, it is quite effective in controlling mild hypertension in combination with a diuretic agent.

Side Effects. The major side effects and complications of reserpine include nasal stuffiness and increased gastric acid secretion, which may occasionally activate an ulcer. The most serious problem, however, is CNS depression, sometimes severe enough to lead to suicide. It has been suggested that severe depression occurs predominantly in intelligent people who engage in sedentary occupations. Although frequent with the larger doses that were prevalent in the past (i.e., 0.75 mg a day), depression is much less common with the currently recommended maximal dose of 0.25 mg a day. Patients with a history of depression should not be given this drug, and all patients should be warned to discontinue reserpine if they begin to feel depressed or if they develop suspicious symptoms such as awakening early in the morning without being able to fall back asleep. Reserpine is contraindicated in patients with peptic ulcer disease and relatively contraindicated in those with Parkinson's disease. Although a possible link between reserpine use and breast cancer was suggested several years ago, subsequent studies have failed to substantiate this association.

Dosage. Reserpine should be prescribed in a dose of 0.125 to 0.25 mg once daily. Larger doses tend to increase the frequency and severity of side effects without providing much additional antihypertensive effect.

Guanethidine (Ismelin)

Guanethidine acts by depleting the reserve pool of norepinephrine and decreasing the amount released when the nerve is stimulated. This interference with norepinephrine release causes a decrease in arteriolar constriction and a modest reduction in peripheral resistance. The blood pressure is somewhat reduced when the patient is in the supine position, but much more so when the patient is standing, since the usual vasoconstrictor response to upright posture is blunted. Guanethidine reduces cardiac output and lowers systolic blood pressure more than diastolic blood pressure. It obviates the increases in heart rate and systolic blood pressure that attend moderate exercise. Since guanethidine works best when patients are upright, the physician should anticipate the occurrence of a postural decline in blood pressure, not just as a side effect of the drug but rather as evidence that a therapeutic effect has been reached. The effects of guanethidine tend to be cumulative over several weeks, perhaps more so in the setting of renal insufficiency.

Side Effects. The major side effect of the drug is postural or exercise-induced hypotension. This complication may be aggravated by any factor that promotes vasodilation, such as alcohol ingestion or a hot environment. Patients should be instructed to avoid this occurrence by such measures as rising slowly from the supine or seated position and wearing good elastic hose. Failure of ejaculation or retrograde ejaculation occurs commonly, but true impotence is rare. Since guanethidine does not cross the blood-brain barrier, there is little if any decrease in the catecholamine content of CNS, and thus sedative or depressant effects do not occur.

Guanethidine is a potent drug, but because, like other Step-4 agents, it has the potential to produce florid side effects (Table 6–10), we fortunately do

TABLE 6–10. PRINCIPAL ADVERSE EFFECTS OF STEP-4 AGENTS GUANETHIDINE, MINOXIDIL, AND CAPTOPRIL

1. Guanethidine
   a. Postural hypotension
   b. Sodium retention
   c. Retrograde ejaculation
2. Minoxidil
   a. Marked sodium retention—prevent with high dose of furosemide
   b. Tachycardia—minimize with beta-blocker, clonidine, or both
   c. Hypertrichosis
   d. Coarsening of facial features
   e. Overly rapid decrement in blood pressure if dose is excessive, or in combination with other medications
3. Captopril
   a. Loss or alteration of taste
   b. Leukopenia; rarely, agranulocytosis
   c. Proteinuria, nephrotic syndrome
   d. Hyperkalemia
   e. Overly rapid decrement in blood pressure if dose is excessive, or in combination with other medications
   f. Reduction in glomerular filtration rate when blood pressure reduction is excessive, or possibly in patients with renal artery stenosis

not have to use this drug except under extraordinary circumstances (i.e., resistance to a multiple-drug regimen).

Dosage. The initial dosage of guanethidine is 10 mg a day, and the dosage should be increased gradually by increments of 10 to 12.5 mg every three to five days.

Methyldopa (Aldomet)

Methyldopa is closely related to the naturally occurring precursor of norepinephrine, dopa, and is incorporated into the biosynthetic pathway within nerve endings. Alpha-methylnorepinephrine is produced from methyldopa, displacing norepinephrine from the stores in the adrenergic nerves as well as in the central nervous system, thus becoming a false transmitter. Although earlier studies suggested that the site of action of methyldopa is in the peripheral adrenergic nerves, more recent studies support a central site of action. It is very likely that multiple mechanisms account for the antihypertensive action of this medication.

The hypotensive action of methyldopa is achieved by a decrease in peripheral resistance, with relatively insignificant effects on cardiac output and heart rate. Since renal vascular resistance may be reduced more than in other vascular beds, GFR and renal blood flow are usually maintained despite the concomitant fall in blood pressure. Although the blood pressure is lowered more in the upright posture than the supine position, significant postural hypotension is not particularly common, because the sympathetic nervous blockade is less complete than that obtaining with guanethidine. Exercise-induced increments in blood pressure are not prevented.

It has been suggested that hypertensive patients with renal insufficiency are particularly sensitive to methyldopa. Such a finding is not attributable to impaired renal excretion of the drug, since serum levels of unconjugated methyldopa have been reported to be lower, not higher, in patients with advanced renal disease.

Side Effects. Somnolence is a common occurrence during the initial few weeks of therapy. A relatively uncommon, albeit potentially serious, adverse effect is hepatotoxicity manifested by fever and abnormal liver function tests. This complication is usually mild and reversible, disappearing when the drug is stopped. If the drug is not discontinued, however, it may rarely lead to severe chronic liver disease; rechallenge may be very hazardous and is contraindicated. Approximately 20 per cent of patients develop a positive direct Coombs' test, but hemolytic anemia occurs in less than 0.5 per cent of patients. Additional side effects include dry mouth and inability to sustain an erection. Finally, a decrease in mental acuity is a troublesome side effect, which often is not fully appreciated until the drug is stopped.

Dosage. Therapy with methyldopa should be started at a dose of 250 mg once or twice a day, and the daily dosage increased to a maximum of 2.0 grams divided into two doses. As mentioned, caution should be exercised in prescribing methyldopa to patients with renal insufficiency; initially the dosage should be halved and care taken to ensure that frank hypotension does not occur.

Clonidine (Catapres)

Clonidine is a potent centrally acting sympatholytic antihypertensive whose principal mode of action is currently believed to involve stimulation of the presynaptic (alpha-2) adrenoceptor. Since this receptor is inhibitory in nature, the result is a decrease in sympathetic outflow from the CNS. As a consequence, with long-term use, there is a normalization of the elevated total peripheral resistance characteristic of essential hypertension without any important depression of cardiac output. A decrease in plasma norepinephrine reflects the sympatholytic activity and correlates with the decrement in blood pressure. There appears to be no chronic suppression of plasma renin activity.

The antihypertensive efficacy of clonidine is similar to that of the other sympatholytic agents such as reserpine, methyldopa, or beta-blockers. Unlike some other adrenergic inhibitors, however, its use does not appear to be associated with renal sodium retention. Perhaps this in part accounts for preliminary data indicating that clonidine may be valuable as a single agent for the management of hypertensive patients. As mentioned elsewhere, clonidine can be used for several special purposes: as acute therapy by oral loading for severe hypertension without crisis, as a substitute for beta-blocker in a regimen requiring the administration of minoxidil, and perhaps in the diagnostic evaluation of some patients suspected of having pheochromocytoma.

Side Effects. The principal side effects of clonidine are dry mouth and sedation. Although these tend to abate after the first several days of use, they are probably partly dose related and sometimes interfere with patient acceptance and compliance. Postural hypotension is not a frequent problem, and sexual dysfunction is said to be less common than that associated with other sympatholytics.

Clonidine, like methyldopa, guanethidine, and propranolol, may rarely unmask (or possibly cause) the "sick sinus syndrome" (also called "bradycardia-tachycardia syndrome"). This condition, which may result in syncope, usually disappears when the medications are withdrawn. The discontinuation syndromes associated with the abrupt withdrawal of clonidine as well as other antihypertensives are discussed below (see Chapter 9).

Dosage. The starting dosage of clonidine is usually 0.1 mg twice daily, and the maximal recommended dosage level ranges from 1.6 to 2.4 mg/day.

Guanabenz (Wytensin)

Guanabenz has recently been marketed in the United States. This guanidine derivative is similar to methyldopa and clonidine in many respects. Guanabenz acts through both central alpha-adrenergic stimulation and peripheral adrenergic neuronal blockage. Preliminary studies suggest that guanabenz may differ from many of the other sympatholytic agents in not causing reactive fluid retention. Indeed, there are fragmentary data to suggest that the drug may have modest natriuretic properties.

Drugs with central sympatholytic action (such as clonidine and methyldopa as well as guanabenz) decrease sympathethic tone but do not inhibit reflex responses as completely as drugs, such as guanethidine, that act peripherally.

Side Effects. Side effects include sedation, dry mouth, and weakness. In analogy with clonidine, sudden cessation of guanabenz therapy may result in withdrawal symptomatology.

Dosage. The initial dose of guanabenz is 4 mg per day, given in a twice-daily regimen. The dosage may be increased in increments of 4 to 8 mg per day every one to two weeks. A maximum daily dosage of 32 mg twice daily should not be exceeded.

Prazosin (Minipress)

Prazosin is one of the more recently marketed antihypertensive medications that can be used either for Step-2 or Step-3. Of interest is the fact that the results of several initial studies were interpreted as indicating a direct vasodilator mode of action for this medication, whereas it is now considered that selective blockade of peripheral postsynaptic (alpha-1) receptor is the primary if not the sole mechanism of action.

Figure 6–5 depicts the sites of action of alpha-blocking drugs on alpha receptors. As can be seen, phentolamine and phenoxybenzamine block both the presynaptic (alpha-2) and postsynaptic (alpha-1) receptor sites. In contrast, prazosin primarily blocks the postsynaptic receptor. Thus prazosin leaves the presynaptic receptor, which modulates an inhibitory pathway, intact. The resultant unaltered activity of the inhibitory pathway has been postulated to account for the absence of prominent tachycardia with the use of this agent.

In a hypertensive patient with a normal heart, prazosin has little effect on cardiac output. On the other hand, by reducing both preload and afterload, it frequently is of substantial benefit in the management of patients with severe chronic congestive heart failure. Although partial tolerance may influence the response to the long-term use of prazosin for this purpose, to date no tolerance has been demonstrated regarding the chronic antihypertensive efficacy. In patients with severe hypertension mandating a Step-3 regimen, the medication works well in combination with beta-blockers and diuretics.

Side Effects. Because it does not act centrally, prazosin has not been associated with mental depression. Another bane of many of the other sympatholytics, sexual dysfunction, does not appear to be caused by this medication. Likewise, since cardiac output is not constrained, prazosin, unlike beta-blockers, does not tend to reduce exercise tolerance. Finally, the drug produces no depression in renal function and does not accentuate bronchospasm or impair carbohydrate or lipid metabolism. Generally, the side effects of prazosin are transient and mild; they include headache, dizziness, drowsiness, weakness and lack of energy, and nausea. Orthostatic hypotension is not a frequent problem, but the physician must be aware of a potential but usually avoidable adverse effect—the so-called first-dose phenomenon. When the medication was first introduced and initial doses greater than 1 mg were used, there were many instances of marked dizziness or even syncope related to severe orthostatic hypotension, which occurred 30 to 90 minutes after ingestion of the medication. The current recommendation, to limit the first dose to 1 mg at bedtime with avoidance of upright posture for at least two hours, has reduced the incidence of this side effect to a very low level (perhaps one in 1000).

Dosage. We recommend that an initial dose of prazosin of 1 mg be taken after assuming supine position at bedtime, followed by 1 mg twice daily. This dosage is ineffective in a large percentage of patients, and the average dose necessary to control blood pressure in patients with moderate to severe hypertension is 8 to 12 mg/day. The maximal dose generally used is between 20 and 30 mg/day.

Pargyline (Eutonyl)

Pargyline is the sole remaining member of the monoamine oxidase (MAO)–inhibitory medications still available in the United States for the treatment of hypertension. Because of the numerous drug interactions with this agent, many of which are serious and even life-threatening, and because of the availability of numerous other antihypertensive agents, we do not believe that pargyline has a role in the management of hypertension today.

PERIPHERAL VASODILATORS

Hydralazine (Apresoline)

Hydralazine is well absorbed from the gut, with maximal blood levels being attained three to four hours following ingestion. The drug acts directly to relax the smooth musculature in the walls of the peripheral arterioles and influences the resistance vessels much more than the capacitance vessels. Consequently, peripheral resistance and blood pressure decrease. The ability of hydralazine to relax vascular smooth muscle is not uniform, so that whereas it tends to increase splanchnic, coronary, cerebral, and renal blood flow, skeletal muscle and skin blood flows are not augmented. These unique effects have important clinical correlates, such as the preservation of renal function in patients with pre-existing renal insufficiency.

Side Effects. As a consequence of hydralazine-induced peripheral vasodilatation, heart rate, stroke volume, cardiac output, and myocardial oxygen requirements all increase. Many patients find the tachycardia, headache, and flushed feeling bothersome. A more worrisome occurrence is the potential for angina in patients with pre-existing coronary artery disease. Although tolerance to these side effects sometimes develops, they sharply limit the value of hydralazine as a sole antihypertensive agent. It appears that these troublesome side effects may be less common in elderly patients or in those previously taking diuretics. They can also be neutralized by combining the medication with one of the sympatholytic agents that blunts the increase in heart rate and cardiac output.

In addition to the tachycardia, palpitations, and headache mentioned above, other side effects include anorexia, nausea, vomiting, diarrhea, and, less commonly, tremor and muscle cramps. Hydralazine-induced lupus erythematosus is very rare if the daily dose is limited to less than 200 to 300 mg and perhaps if the total dose administered is restricted to less than 100 grams.

Clinical Use and Dosage. Whereas in the past hydralazine was used extensively as a second-choice agent, its side effects—reflex tachycardia and sodium and fluid retention (both of which tend to offset its antihypertensive properties)—make it an excellent Step-3 medication. This is because when hydralazine is combined with a diuretic and sympatholytic agent, both the side effects and the "pseudotolerance" are obviated and an additive antihypertensive effect is observed.

In order to lessen initial side effects, therapy with hydralazine should be started at doses that are frequently suboptimal, i.e., 25 mg twice daily; subsequently this may be gradually increased to a maximum dose of 300 mg daily. Beyond this level, approximately 10 per cent of patients develop a lupus-like syndrome.

Hydralazine should be administered with caution or perhaps even avoided in patients with symptomatic coronary artery disease. If used, it should be prescribed in conjunction with a beta-blocker. Similarly, in light of its ability to increase cerebral blood flow, hydralazine should probably be avoided in patients with recent cerebral hemorrhage.

Minoxidil

Minoxidil is an orally administered direct vasodilator that is not only much more potent than hydralazine, the only other currently available medication of this type, but also one of the most potent antihypertensive agents of any class. If used in sufficient dosage, it is frequently effective in patients whose severe hypertension has been resistant to other antihypertensive medications used in combination, including the angiotensin-converting enzyme inhibitor, captopril.

Aside from its potency, additional advantages of minoxidil include a rapid onset of action of approximately 30 minutes, a maximum effect within two to three hours, and a total duration of action exceeding 24 hours, which allows a once-daily dosing regimen. Furthermore, its long-term use has not been associated with true tolerance, although pseudotolerance related to the retention of dietary sodium may occur. Finally, since the drug does not act centrally and affects primarily the resistance vessels (arterioles), its use is associated neither with CNS side effects, such as sedation, nor with postural hypotension.

Side Effects. As is the case with the other Step-4 agents (Table 6–10), the potential for important adverse effects (together with its striking blood pressure–lowering action) accounts for the current recommendation to limit the use of minoxidil to patients manifesting severe resistant hypertension with evidence of end-organ dysfunction. One of the most striking side effects is the induction of sodium retention, which probably results from the combined effects of reduction in blood pressure, renal vasodilatation, and activation of the renin-angiotensin-aldosterone axis. If this sodium-retaining tendency is not obviated, it is not unusual for patients to gain as much as 10 to 15 pounds or more in the first week of therapy. This may result in massive edema, impaired blood pressure response, and congestive heart failure. As is the case with hydralazine, unless prevented by concurrent use of sympatholytic agents, minoxidil may induce tachycardia and increased cardiac work (with the potential for aggravation of the symptoms of ischemic heart disease).

Two other major side effects are excessive hair growth and pericardial effusion. The former occurs in both men and women and, not surprisingly, is particularly distressing to the latter. The hypertrichosis is generalized and often includes the face and upper extremities. It typically regresses several weeks after discontinuation of the medication and can be controlled by depilatories. Pericardial effusion is an infrequent occurrence, but one that can sometimes be of great import because it carries the risk of cardiac tamponade. Although it tends to occur in patients with a particular tendency to develop fluid accumulations in serosal cavities (i.e., those with renal failure, congestive heart failure, or both), it may appear in the absence of apparent predisposing factors. The effusions may or may not respond to an increased dosage of diuretic and usually regress upon discontinuation of the medication. Finally, because of its potent antihypertensive effect, minoxidil administration may initially be associated with dramatic decrements in renal function in those patients with pre-existing renal impairment. Later, particularly if the baseline serum creatinine level is less than 4 mg/dl, renal function frequently returns to or exceeds the baseline value.

Clinical Use of Minoxidil. Because of the above-mentioned potency and side effects, the current use of minoxidil is limited. Nevertheless, it is an extremely valuable agent in patients with resistant hypertension and has permitted control of the blood pressure with a reasonably simple regimen in many patients who had been poorly controlled despite the use of three or even four potent agents. It may be that future studies will show that very low dose administration of minoxidil will provide excellent and safe control of the blood pressure in patients with moderate or even mild hypertension, but such information is not now at hand.

The use of minoxidil should be supervised by an experienced physician. With occasional exceptions we prefer to initiate treatment with minoxidil in hospitalized patients to allow rapid recognition of the unusual patient who develops excessive decrements in blood pressure. After the patient is discharged on an appropriate dose of minoxidil, it is imperative that the physician clearly outline the patient's role in the avoidance of one of the major side effects of this drug, sodium retention. The patient should be instructed how best to restrict his sodium intake. Furthermore, he should check his weight daily and monitor his blood pressure at home, if feasible. Important changes in body weight or blood pressure should be reported immediately to the physician to allow appropriate adjustment of the dose of his medications or to permit an immediate evaluation if necessary. In the patient with underlying renal insufficiency, laboratory surveillance is essential.

Minoxidil should be given in association with high dosages of a potent diuretic such as furosemide (usually 80 to 160 mg or more) and with limitation of dietary sodium intake. In addition, either a beta-adrenoceptor blocker or clonidine must be given coterminously to prevent tachycardia and to complement the antihypertensive action. Of interest, in countries where calcium entry blockers are widely used for the treatment of hypertension, they appear to have supplanted minoxidil in the management of patients with severe hypertension.

INHIBITORS OF THE RENIN-ANGIOTENSIN SYSTEM

At present, there are several available approaches to reduce the activity of the renin-angiotensin system in man. Until recently, the most widely used approach has been to reduce renin release and hence lower PRA, as for example by the administration of beta-blockers. A second approach is to administer a competitive antagonist that attaches to angiotensin receptors but does not duplicate its cellular effects. An example of such an antagonist is saralasin. The third and perhaps the most promising approach consists of the use of an agent such as captopril that inhibits the conversion of inactive angiotensin I to active angiotensin II.

Saralasin

Saralasin is a recently marketed analogue of angiotensin II that competes for angiotensin II receptors in blood vessels and other tissues and blocks the response to exogenous angiotensin I and angiotensin II in a dose-dependent fashion.

Since it has been proposed as a diagnostic tool both to identify patients with renovascular hypertension and to predict the outcome of surgery, it will be discussed in greater detail in Chapter 14.

Captopril

The prototype of the converting enzyme inhibitors is captopril. Although captopril was primarily introduced for use as a Step-4 agent in patients resistant to other antihypertensive agents, preliminary data suggest that in low doses it is effective and well tolerated in patients with mild hypertension.

There are several mechanisms whereby captopril may lower the blood pressure. Most evidence suggests that the blood pressure–lowering effect is attributable to a reduction of the level of circulating angiotensin II, although some observers have failed to find a close correlation between PRA levels and the subsequent blood pressure response. It is worthwhile pointing out that as a consequence of angiotensin II reduction, PRA (which is an index of angiotensin I) increases. This phenomenon should not concern the clinician, since it is angiotensin II and not PRA that modulates the increase in blood pressure. It is possible that the antihypertensive action of captopril may be attributable in part to a potentiation of the vasodilator substance bradykinin by the prevention of its breakdown. In addition, because of the interrelationship between angiotensin II and catecholamines, it is possible that captopril tones down the sympathetic nervous system, which accounts for the low incidence of tachycardia. Finally, there is evidence to suggest that the ability of captopril to stimulate prostaglandin synthesis may contribute to its antihypertensive effect.

Regardless of mechanism, the major action of captopril is to lower blood pressure, primarily by reducing peripheral resistance. Cardiac output and heart rate change little in the patient with a normal heart, whereas the patient with heart failure may be benefited by a reduction in both preload and afterload. In contrast to many other nondiuretic antihypertensive agents, captopril does not cause volume expansion, probably because of its inhibition of aldosterone secretion and perhaps its ability to augment GFR and renal blood flow.

A new converting enzyme inhibitor soon to be marketed is called enalapril. In contrast to captopril, it lacks the sulfydryl group that has been postulated to account for some of the observed side effects associated with the administration of this class of medication.

Side Effects (Table 6–10). Approximately 20 per cent of patients receiving captopril develop a skin rash or some disturbance of taste. In the majority of instances, these side effects are relatively mild and may disappear, even with continuation of captopril administration. Loss of taste, however, which is assumed to occur as a result of the binding of captopril to zinc ions, may give rise to significant weight loss.

A more serious, albeit rare, complication is the development of membranous glomerulopathy, which occurs in about 1 per cent of patients taking captopril and manifests initially with proteinuria. It should be pointed out, however, that there is no consensus regarding the subject, and some observers have even questioned the existence of this entity. It is thought that the glomerulopathy is attributable to the binding of heavy metals by the free sulfhydryl moiety in captopril, analogous to the glomerulopathy seen with other drugs with sulfhydryl moieties, such as penicillamine. Finally, a rare, albeit serious, complication is bone marrow suppression. This complication may present as leukopenia or agranulocytosis and has rarely proven to be fatal. If it occurs, the drug should be withdrawn, and the patient should not be rechallenged with captopril. Although the hematologic and renal side effects of captopril do not occur as frequently as was feared when the medication was first introduced, we believe that the clinician treating a patient with captopril should monitor the white blood cell count and urinary protein level every two to three months.

Hyperkalemia, which is of sufficient magnitude to be clinically worrisome, may occur in patients with diminished renal reserve or disordered internal potassium homeostasis. Although the lessening of urinary potassium loss seen with captopril is usually beneficial, countering the hypokalemia induced by diuretics, on occasion it may provoke hyperkalemia in patients whose ability to excrete potassium is already impaired (i.e., by renal failure, concomitant use of potassium-sparing diuretics, etc.; see pp. 78–81).

A recently recognized phenomenon is the apparent potential for captopril-induced functional renal insufficiency in patients with bilateral renal artery stenosis (or possibly when renal artery stenosis occurs in a patient with a single kidney). In hypertensive patients without renal artery stenosis, the administration of captopril is not associated with a decrement in renal function, unless the reduction in blood pressure is too great. On the other hand, it appears that in the presence of renal artery stenosis, the adaptive intrarenal mechanisms to support the GFR are dependent, at least in part, on vasoconstriction of the postglomerular (efferent) arteriole by angiotensin II. Blockade of the RAA axis by captopril seems to obviate this protective adaptation and may result in a considerable fall in GFR, which is reversed when the medication is discontinued.

Clinical Use and Dosage. The appropriate setting in which to initiate captopril therapy is not established. Although not every patient should be hospitalized before beginning captopril therapy, this should be a consideration in many patients because of the possibility of hypotension. If captopril therapy is begun in an outpatient setting, the "test dose" approach has particular merit. The patient should be seated and given a dose of either 6.25 or 12.5 mg. The blood pressure is monitored at 10 to 15 minute intervals for the subsequent hour. At that time, if there are no untoward effects, the patient may be sent home. In the elderly patient, or in a patient concomitantly receiving other medications, the test dose should be 6.25 mg.

The manufacturer suggests that all other antihypertensive medications be discontinued before initiation of captopril therapy. In practice, this is difficult to achieve, because such patients have severe hypertension, which will not permit an abrupt discontinuation of therapy. In many such patients, it is more prudent to continue the other medications in reduced doses and to begin captopril in smaller than usual doses (i.e., 6.25 or 12.5 mg, by dividing the scored captopril tablet).

Adding Captopril to Existing Regimen. An often-asked question is exactly how to add captopril to the existing multidrug regimen of a patient with severe hypertension. Obviously, the method must differ somewhat in each patient. In order to provide a guideline for the approach to this problem, we would like to cite the following example of what we recommended recently in a hospitalized patient whose blood pressure was 175/115 mm Hg in spite of compliance with a regimen consisting of chlorthalidone, 50 mg once a day; propranolol, 160 mg twice a day; and hydralazine, 100 mg twice a day:

1. Hold hydralazine if the diastolic pressure is less than 110 mm Hg, but continue the beta-blocker and diuretic at the pre-existing doses.
2. Administer either 6.25 or 12.5 mg of captopril in the morning, two hours after breakfast.
3. After this test dose, monitor the blood pressure every 15 minutes for the first hour, then every 30 minutes for the next two to four hours, depending on the blood pressure.
4. Keep patient supine for the first two hours after the test dose.
5. If, 12 hours after the first dose, the blood pressure is greater than 140/85 mm Hg, give 25 mg of captopril. If the blood pressure is not frankly low but is less than 140/85 mm Hg, repeat the test dose.
6. Beginning on day 2, if blood pressure is not low, change the captopril dose to 25 mg three times a day.
7. After the appropriate captopril dosage has been determined, taper the dose of the beta-blocker (if the blood pressure is well controlled).
8. Monitor the patient for alterations of renal function or serum electrolytes (i.e., azotemia, hyperkalemia).

If the "test dose" method is not used, then the standard initial dose of captopril is 25 mg three times a day, taken one hour before or two hours after meals. If a satisfactory reduction of blood pressure has not been achieved after one or two weeks, the dose may be increased to 50 mg three times a day. If the blood pressure still is not controlled satisfactorily, a diuretic should be added to the regimen. Occasional patients may require an increase in dosage to 100 mg or 150 mg three times a day. A maximum daily dosage of 450 mg of captopril should not be exceeded. Of interest, recent preliminary reports suggest that the optimal dose of captopril in hypertension may be considerably less than previously supposed. Investigators in London have proposed that as little as 25 mg three times a day may provide as much blood pressure–lowering effect as much larger doses, with less potential for adverse efects. If captopril and diuretics together do not suffice, the cautious addition of a beta-blocker is warranted.

In light of the frequent coexistence of hypertension and diabetes, it should be mentioned that captopril has been reported to produce a false positive urinary test for ketones.

Because of captopril's limited use to date in the United States, its great potency, and its potentially important adverse side effects, we believe that the manufacturer's current recommendation for its use—that is, that the prescription of the medication be limited to the patient with severe hypertension not responsive to the classic Step-Care approach—is reasonable. As was mentioned to be the case for minoxidil, it is not unlikely that captopril may prove to be an excellent agent for the management (perhaps as a single medication) of moderate or even mild hypertension, but data sufficient to recommend such an approach are not yet available. Of interest, preliminary data indicate that captopril, in analogy with the beta-blockers, might be less effective in black patients than in white ones.

Recently, Laragh and his associates have proposed that converting enzyme inhibitors may have a role in dictating the choice of an antihypertensive regimen in patients with essential hypertension. They utilize the antihypertensive response to a single dose of captopril as a guide for determining the initial choice of an antihypertensive agent. Attractive as such an approach appears to be, it seems to be marred by a substantial number of false positive and negative responses. It should be noted that a minority of patients who ultimately will respond to captopril therapy will not do so in the first few days following initiation of therapy. This is one reason that using the response to a single dose of captopril to determine the selection of a hypertension regimen may be misleading.

CALCIUM-ENTRY BLOCKERS

Since increased levels of intracellular calcium induce vascular smooth muscle contraction, and since alterations in cellular calcium may be involved in the pathogenesis of essential hypertension, attention has focused recently on the antihypertensive properties of drugs that block the cellular entry of calcium.

Although originally termed calcium-channel blockers or calcium antagonists, the more appropriate designation is calcium-entry blocker or calcium ion influx inhibitor. It should be emphasized that these drugs are not pharmacologic antagonists of calcium. Rather, they inhibit the transmembrane influx of calcium ions into cardiac and smooth muscle cells but do not compete with calcium for intracellular target sites. They do not change serum calcium concentration.

These medications include a very heterogeneous group of compounds, both in chemical structure and tissue specificity. One drug may have much more effect than another on small arterioles. For example, nifedipine appears to be a much more potent arteriolar vasodilator but has fewer cardiac effects

TABLE 6–11. DIFFERING CARDIOVASCULAR EFFECTS OF CALCIUM-ENTRY BLOCKERS

Drug	Heart Rate	A-V Conduction	Blood Pressure
Nifedipine	↑	→	↓↓
Verapamil	↓ or ↓↓	↓↓	↓
Diltiazem	↓	↓	↓

↑ = increase; ↓ = decrease; → = no change; two arrows indicate a greater quantitative change.

than verapamil. Thus, it reduces systemic peripheral resistance to a greater degree. Additionally, the effect of these agents on veins may differ from one vein to another and also from one drug to another. Table 6–11 summarizes the differing effects of the three available calcium-entry blockers on heart rate, A-V conduction, and blood pressure. As can be seen, nifedipine appears to be the most effective blood pressure–lowering agent. It also is the one that consistently increases the heart rate but has the least influence on A-V conduction and sinus node recovery time, and thus it can often be used together with a beta-blocker. The clinical relevance of these pharmacologic differences is that calcium-entry blockers, because of their differing vascular and cardiac effects, are not interchangeable.

Calcium-entry blockers lower the blood pressure of hypertensive patients by reducing peripheral resistance. Since many of these agents also reduce the venous return to the heart by vasodilation of the splanchnic veins, the reduction of blood pressure may be associated with relatively little increase in cardiac output or heart rate. The net cardiac effect of the entry blockers is the result of many actions. On one hand, the direct effect is to depress cardiac performance (negative inotropy). Nevertheless, in the hypertensive patient, by reducing blood pressure they improve cardiac function. Reflex stimulation of the sympathetic nervous system should also tend to support cardiac function.

In summary, a patient with relatively good left ventricular function can be treated with a calcium-entry blocker. If need be, a beta-blocker can be added to reduce excessive tachycardia or to provide additive antihypertensive action. Although this combination might be dangerous for a patient with marked ventricular dysfunction, most experts experienced with such regimens have been impressed with their safety.

An interesting aspect of this class of antihypertensive medications is their atypical action on renal sodium handling. In contrast to many other nondiuretic antihypertensive drugs, the direct renal effect of calcium-entry blockers appears to be facilitated sodium excretion. Nevertheless, their net effect on sodium homeostasis is determined by the sum of the effects on blood pressure, cardiac performance, systemic vascular resistance, and renal tubular transport.

Side Effects. As with other potent antihypertensive agents, an excessive decrement in blood pressure is possible when calcium-entry blockers are used. This tends to occur during initial titration or at the time of subsequent upward dosage adjustment and may be more likely in patients receiving beta-blockers coterminously. Occasional patients with underlying coronary artery disease develop increased frequency, duration, or severity of angina when starting or increasing the dose of nifedipine. Likewise, nifedipine may exacerbate the increased angina associated with abrupt discontinuation of beta-blocker therapy. Congestive heart failure is a rare complication, theoretically more likely in a patient with aortic stenosis. An important common side effect of nifedipine is peripheral edema. Typically, this relates to arteriolar vasodilation rather than to left ventricular dysfunction. It occurs in about 10 per cent of patients, primarily involves the lower extremities, and usually is corrected by the administration of a diuretic. Other side effects include dizziness, flushing, and, rarely, muscle cramps or tremor, diarrhea, constipation, and anxiety. As expected, some of the side effects are dose related, particularly hypotension and peripheral edema. Finally, nifedipine and verapamil have been reported to increase serum digoxin levels, presumably by decreasing renal and metabolic clearance.

Dosage. None of the calcium-entry blockers has been approved yet in the United States for the indication of hypertension. Thus, although no exact recommendation for dosage can be made, the available experience from Europe with nifedipine suggests that the effective dose for blood pressure lowering may be in the range of approximately 20 to 40 mg/day in divided doses.

Although at present only nifedipine is being extensively used to treat hypertension, it is likely that in the next several years additional calcium-entry blockers will become available.

SEXUAL SIDE EFFECTS OF THE ANTIHYPERTENSIVE DRUGS

The sexual side effects of antihypertensive medications often constitute important problems that complicate the successful control of blood pressure. This topic has recently attracted much attention in both the medical and lay press. Sexual effects loom important by contributing to poor compliance and treatment dropout, and they may even lead to failure to seek treatment. A patient's lack of understanding of the cause of the sexual dysfunction, or misunderstanding of its nature, may adversely affect his or her interpersonal relationships.

Antihypertensive medications, particularly those acting directly on the sympathetic nervous system, are prone to interfere with sexual activity and performance. Although some reported sexual side effects are psychosomatic, controlled clinical studies have documented statistically significant relationships between antihypertensive drugs and sexual dysfunction. In one such study of 7513 male patients with mild hypertension, the incidence of impotence was six times higher in those treated with the beta blocker propranolol than in those who received a placebo.

Most reports focus on male sexual dysfunction, at least in part because the problem is more readily apparent in men than in women. The physician, however, should be aware of these side effects in women as well. Table 6–12 summarizes sexual and reproductive side effects for both sexes and shows the implicated agents. For example, reserpine has been linked not only to decreased libido and impotence but to ejaculatory and orgasmic difficulties. Because of its potential side effects it is used less often today and should be prescribed with special caution.

Since it is clear that antihypertensive medications commonly produce diverse sexual side effects, what should the physician do when confronted with the problem? First, the clinician should accept the report of sexual dysfunction matter-of-factly. We do not recommend an excessive questioning of the patient that connotes a challenge of the complaint. We may be remiss in dismissing the patient's complaint on the basis of being unable to formulate a likely mechanism for the reported side effect. For example, recent evidence has

TABLE 6–12.   SEXUAL AND REPRODUCTIVE SIDE EFFECTS OF COMMONLY USED ANTIHYPERTENSIVE AGENTS

Side Effect	Medication
WOMEN	
Breast enlargement, tenderness, or both	Clonidine, methyldopa, spironolactone
Loss of or decrease in libido	Diuretics, guanethidine, methyldopa, propranolol, reserpine
Reduction of vaginal lubrication	Diuretics
Menstrual irregularities and impaired ovulation	Spironolactone
MEN	
Loss of or decrease in libido	Diuretics, guanethidine, methyldopa, propranolol, reserpine
Impotence	Most antihypertensive agents
Ejaculatory abnormalities	Clonidine, guanethidine, methyldopa, reserpine
Gynecomastia, breast tenderness, or both	Spironolactone, methyldopa, clonidine

confirmed earlier reports that drugs, such as thiazide-type diuretics, that ostensibly do not alter autonomic function may indeed induce impotence.

Because of the propensity of antihypertensive agents to cause sexual dysfunction, the physician should assume initially that the therapy may indeed be at fault and direct efforts toward the twin goals of eliminating or reducing the severity of the side effect while maintaining effective control of the blood pressure. The physician should project confidence that both of these goals can be fulfilled. In our experience, manipulation of the drug regimen is usually successful, with the caveat that organic nondrug-related impotence is common.

COMBINATION ANTIHYPERTENSIVE MEDICATIONS

There is an abundance of antihypertensive combination medications available for the management of the hypertensive patient, and these are listed in Appendix 3. What should the approach of the clinician be to the use of a combination preparation? We believe that a dogmatic denigration of combination regimens is not in order. Although there are clear-cut drawbacks to the use of such fixed-dose combinations, their use is acceptable and perhaps even desirable in selected patients. The clinician should determine that the individual agents of the combination are efficacious and free of important side effects and that the combination can provide a dosage of each similar to that previously observed to be appropriate when the components were used separately. In this case, a combination medication may offer the advantage of simplicity, and may consequently improve compliance. Furthermore, there may be a cost advantage to the patient of using a combination tablet rather than the components as separate tablets. Of note, the WHO, in its recent recommendations for patients with mild hypertension, points out that, for the above-mentioned reasons, drugs in a single tablet or capsule often constitute the treatment of choice once the need for two drugs has been established.

REFERENCES

Freis, ED: The Modern Management of Hypertension. Veterans Administration (0–560–021), Washington, DC, 1974.

Tarazi, RC: Long-term effective antihypertensive therapy. Ann Intern Med 93:771–772, 1980.

Editorial: Twenty-four-hour blood-pressure control: does it matter? Lancet I:222–223, 1983.

Kaplan, HR, and Smith RD: Antihypertensive drugs: proposed sites and mechanisms of action. Fed Proc 40:2268–2274, 1981.

Anderson RJ, and Kirk, LM: Methods of improving patient compliance in chronic disease states. Arch Intern Med 142:1673–1675, 1982.

Diuretics

Anderson, J, Godfrey, BE, Hill, DM, Munro-Faure, AD, and Sheldon, J: A comparison of the effects of hydrochlorothiazide and of furosemide in the treatment of hypertensive patients. QJ Med 40:541–560, 1971.

Holland, OB, Gomez-Sanchez, CE, Kuhnert, LV, Poindexter, C, Pak, YC: Antihypertensive comparison of furosemide with hydrochlorothiazide for black patients. Arch Intern Med 139:1015–1021, 1979.

Murphy, MB, Lewis, PJ, Kohner, E, Schumer, B, and Dollery, CT: Glucose intolerance in hypertensive patients treated with diuretics; a fourteen-year follow-up. Lancet II: 1293–1295, 1982.

Berglund, G., and Andersson, O: Beta-blockers or diuretics in hypertension? A six year follow-up of blood pressure and metabolic side effects. Lancet I:744–747, 1981.

Medical Research Council Working Party on Mild to Moderate Hypertension. Adverse reactions to bendrofluazide and propranolol for the treatment of mild hypertension. Lancet II:539–543, 1981.

Sandor, FF, Pickens, PT, and Crallan, J: Variations of plasma potassium concentrations during long-term treatment of hypertension with diuretics without potassium supplements. Br Med J 284:711–715, 1982.

Kassirer, JP, and Harrington, JT: Diuretics and potassium metabolism: A reassessment of the need, effectiveness and safety of potassium therapy. Kidney Int. 11:505–515, 1977.

Harrington, JT, Isner, JM, and Kassirer, JP: Our national obsession with potassium. Am J Med 73:155–159, 1982.

Holland, OB, Nixon, JV, and Kuhnert, L: Diuretic-induced ventricular ectopic activity. Am J Med 70:762–768, 1981.

Hollifield, JW, and Slaton, PE: Thiazide diuretics, hypokalemia and cardiac arrhythmias. Acta Med Scand Suppl 647:67–73, 1980.

Solomon, RJ, and Cole, AG: Importance of potassium in patients with acute myocardial infarction. Acta Med Scand Suppl 647:87–93, 1980.

Dyckner, T, and Wester, PO: Relation between potassium, magnesium and cardiac arrhythmias. Acta Med Scand Suppl 647:163–169, 1980.

Wester, PO, and Dyckner, T: Diuretic treatment and magnesium losses. Acta Med Scand Suppl 647:145–152, 1980.

McMahon, FG, Ryan, JR, Akdamar, K, and Ertan, A: Upper gastrointestinal lesions after potassium chloride supplements: a controlled clinical trial. Lancet II:1059–1061, 1982.

Fichman, MP, Vorherr, H, Kleeman, CR, and Telfer, N: Diuretic-induced hyponatremia. Ann Intern Med 75:853–863, 1971.

Friedman R, and Flamenbaum, W: Pharmacology, therapeutic efficacy, and adverse effects of bumetanide, a new "loop" diuretic. Pharmacotherapy 2:213–221, 1982.

Ram, CV, Garrett, BN, and Kaplan, NM: Moderate sodium restriction and various diuretics in the treatment of hypertension. Arch Intern Med 141:1015–1019, 1981.

Cockcroft, DW, and Gault, MH: Prediction of creatinine clearance from serum creatinine. Nephron 16:31–41, 1976.

Beta-Adrenoceptor Blocking Agents

Frishmann, WH: Beta-adrenergic blockade in clinical practice. Hosp Prac, pp 57–58, Sept 1982.

Frishman, WH: Recent advances in beta-adrenoceptor blocker pharmacology. Am Heart Assoc Council Clin Cardiol 9:1–17, 1983.

Man In't Veld, AJ, and Schalekamp, MADH: How intrinsic sympathomimetic activity modulates the haemodynamic responses to beta-adrenoreceptor antagonists. A clue to the nature of their antihypertensive mechanism. Br J Clin Pharmacol 13:245S–257S, 1982.

Kirkendall, WM (guest ed.): Proceedings of an International Symposium on Pindolol. Am Heart J 104:333–520, 1982.

Plotnick, GD, Fisher, ML, Hamilton, JH, and Hamilton, BP: Intrinsic sympathomimetic activity of pindolol. Evidence for interaction with pretreatment sympathetic tone. Am J Med 74:625–629, 1983.

Bolli, P, Bühler, FR, Raeder, EA, Amann, FW, Meier, M, Rogg, H, and Burckhardt, D: Lack of beta-adrenoreceptor hypersensitivity after abrupt withdrawal of long-term therapy with oxprenolol. Circulation 64:1130–1134, 1981.

Taylor, SH, Silke, B, and Lee, PS: Intravenous beta-blockade in coronary heart disease. Is cardioselectivity or intrinsic sympathomimetic activity hemodynamically useful? N Engl J Med 306:631–635, 1982.

Braunwald, E, Muller, JE, Kloner, RA, and Maroko, PR: Role of beta-adrenergic blockade in the therapy of patients with myocardial infarction. Am J Med 74:113–123, 1983.

Epstein, M, and Oster, JR: Beta-blockers and the kidney. Mineral Electrolyte Metabolism 8:237–254, 1982.

Other Inhibitors of the Sympathetic Nervous System

Louis, WJ, Taylor, H, McNeil, JJ, Jarrott, B, and Rand, MJ: Clinical pharmacology of adrenergic-adrenoreceptor-blocking drugs. Am Heart J 104:407–412, 1982.

Sambhi, MP, and Villarreal, H (guest eds.): Central alpha-adrenoceptors: clinical applications in cardiovascular disease. Chest 83 (Suppl):293–440, 1983.

Drayer, JIM, and Weber, MA: Amtihypertensive agents which inhibit sympathetic activity: potentially adverse effects of combination treatment. Am Heart J 104:660–664, 1982.

Itskovitz, HD (guest ed.): Long-term treatment of hypertension with methyldopa. A retrospective multiclinic study. J Cardiovas Pharmacol 3:S75–S120, 1981.

Fouad, FM, Nakashima, Y, Tarazi, RC, and Salcedo, EE: Reversal of left ventricular hypertrophy in hypertensive patients treated with methyldopa. Lack of association with blood pressure control. Am J Cardiol 49:795–801, 1982.

Lowenstein J: Clonidine. Ann Intern Med 92:74–77, 1980.

Supplement on Clonidine: J Cardiovas Pharmacol 2(Suppl 1):S1–S89, 1980.

Robertson, D, Goldberg, MR, Hollister, AS, Wade, D, and Robertson, RM: Clonidine raises blood pressure in severe idiopathic orthostatic hypotension. Am J Med 74:193–200, 1983.

Brogden, RN, Heel, RC, Speight, TM, and Avery, GS: Prazosin: a review of its pharmacological properties and therapeutic efficacy in hypertension. Drugs 14:163–197, 1977.

Lowenstein, J, and Steele, JM, Jr: Prazosin: mechanism of action and role in antihypertensive therapy. Cardiovasc Med 4:885–891, 1979.

Colucci, WS: Alpha-adrenergic receptor blockade with prazosin. Ann Intern Med 97:66–77, 1982.

Vasodilators

Linas, SL, and Nies, AS: Minoxidil. Ann Intern Med 94:61–65, 1981.

Perry, HM, Jr: Minoxidil and improvement of renal function in uremic malignant hypertension. Ann Intern Med 93:769–771, 1980.

Inhibitors of the Renin-Angiotensin System

Case, DB, Atlas, SA, Laragh, JH, Sealey, JE, Sullivan, PA, and McKinstry, DN: Clinical experience with blockade of the renin-angiotensin-aldosterone system by an oral converting-enzyme inhibitor (SQ 14,225, captopril) in hypertensive patients. Prog Cardiovas Dis 21:195–206, 1978.

Heel, RC, Brogden, RN, Speight, TM, and Avery, GS: Captopril: a preliminary review of its pharmacological properties and therapeutic efficacy. Drugs 20:409–452, 1980.

Zanchetti, A, and Tarazi, RC (guest eds.): Symposium on angiotensin-converting enzyme inhibition: A developing concept. Am J Cardiol 49:1381–1579, 1982.

Smith, SJ, Markandu, ND, and MacGregor, GA: Optimal dose of captopril in hypertension. Lancet II:1460, 1982.

Ferguson, RK, Rothmensch, HH, and Vlasses, PH: Clinical use of captopril. Illustrative cases. JAMA 247:2117–2119, 1983.

Textor, SC, Gephardt, GN, Bravo, EL, Tarazi, RC, Fouad, FM, Tubbs, R, and McMahon, JT: Membranous glomerulopathy associated with captopril therapy. Am J Med 74:705–712, 1983.

Calcium-Entry Blockers

Olivari, MT, Bartorelli, C, Polese, A, Fiorentini, C, Moruzzi, P, and Guazzi, MD: Treatment of hypertension with nifedipine a calcium antagonistic agent. Circulation 59:1056–1062, 1979.

Stone, PH, Antman, EM, Muller, JE, and Braunwald, E: Calcium channel blocking agents in the treatment of cardiovascular disorders. Part II. Hemodynamic effects and clinical applications. Ann Intern Med 93:886–904, 1980.

Editorial: Calcium antagonists in hypertension. Lancet II: 307–308, 1982.

Opie, LH, Lee, L, and White, D: Antihypertensive effects of nifedipine combined with cardioselective beta-adrenergic receptor antagonism by atenolol. Am Heart J 104:606–612, 1982.

Eggertsen, R, and Hansson, L: Effects of treatment with nifedipine and metoprolol in essential hypertension. Eur J Clin Pharmacol 21:389–390, 1982.

McLeay, RAB, Stallard, TJ, Watson, RDS, and Littler, WA: The effect of nifedipine on arterial pressure and reflex cardiac control. Circulation 67:1084–1090, 1983.

Diltiazem for angina pectoris. Med Lett Drugs and Ther 25(629):17–18, 1983.

Safar, ME, Simon, AC, Levenson, JA, and Cazor, JL: Hemodynamic effects of diltiazem in hypertension. Circ Res 52: (Suppl I) 169–173, 1983.

Klein, W, Brandt, D, Vrecko, K, and Harringer, M: Role of calcium antagonists in the treatment of essential hypertension. Circ Res 52: (Suppl I) 174–181, 1983.

Sexual Side Effects of Antihypertensive Agents

Wartman, SA: Sexual side-effects of antihypertensive drugs. Treatment strategies and strictures. Postgrad Med 73:133–138, 1983.

7

DRUG INTERACTIONS IN THE HYPERTENSIVE PATIENT

There are myriad interactions between antihypertensive medications and the other drugs that patients with hypertension commonly receive (Table 7–1). Thus, it has become impossible for any clinician, no matter how astute, to be cognizant of all of them; he must have recourse to a detailed table such as Table 7–1 or to a compendium of such drug interactions. Nevertheless, it is worthwhile to remember the general categories of interactions.

Drug-Drug Interactions

1. Interactions that Alter the Blood Pressure. A common example is a blunting of the antihypertensive action of a medication by another drug. This is typified by the concomitant administration of tricyclic antidepressants and either guanethidine or clonidine. Even worse, indeed potentially life threatening, is the hypertensive crisis induced by concomitant administration of monoamine oxidase (MAO) inhibitors and certain medications, including levodopa. The converse situation is the potentiation of the blood pressure–lowering effect of propranolol by chlorpromazine.

2. Interactions that Alter the Toxicity of One or Both Agents. In addition to interactions that complicate blood pressure control, there are others that do not alter blood pressure but that produce or exacerbate the toxicity of one or the other of the two drugs. An example of this is the potentiation of aminoglycoside-related ototoxicity by the potent loop-type diuretic ethacrynic acid.

3. Interactions that Cause Metabolic or Renal Problems. Another category of interactions (that may overlap Group 2 above) relates to the induction or worsening of metabolic or renal effects. An example of the former is the prolongation of the hypoglycemic effect of insulin by propranolol. An example of the latter is the renal retention of lithium by thiazide-like diuretics.

TABLE 7–1. DRUG INTERACTIONS INVOLVING ANTIHYPERTENSIVE AGENTS

Interacting Drugs	Adverse Effect	Probable Mechanism
General anesthetics with		
Antihypertensives	Hypotension	Usually additive
Nonsteroidal anti-inflammatory agents with		
Diuretics	Decreased natriuresis	Prostaglandin inhibition
Antihypertensives	Decreased BP lowering	Prostaglandin inhibition
K supplements, K-sparing diuretics, beta-blockers	Increased risk of hyperkalemia in predisposed patients	Prostaglandin inhibition
Clonidine with		
Tricyclic antidepressants	Decreased BP lowering	Incompletely defined
Insulin, oral hypoglycemics	Masked symptoms of hypoglycemia	Inhibited catecholamine response
Levodopa	Decreased levodopa effect	Not defined
Tolazoline	Decreased BP lowering	Antagonism at central presynaptic alpha receptor
Propranolol	Increased risk of discontinuation syndrome if clonidine abruptly stopped	Unopposed alpha stimulation
Sympathomimetic amines	Decreased BP lowering	Antagonistic effect
Nitroprusside	Hypotension	Not defined
Diazoxide with		
Phenytoin	Decreased anticonvulsant effect	Not defined
Ethacrynic acid with		
Aminoglycoside antibiotics	Increased ototoxicity	Additive
Furosemide with		
Phenytoin	Decreased diuresis	Not defined
Beta-blocker	Increased beta-blockade	Not defined
Chloral hydrate	Vasomotor instability	Not defined
Guanethidine with		
Tricyclic antidepressants	Decreased BP lowering	Inhibition of uptake of guanethidine at effector site
Oral contraceptives	Decreased BP lowering	Not defined
Phenothiazines	Decreased BP lowering	Inhibition of uptake of guanethidine at effector site
Amphetamine	Decreased BP lowering	Antagonism
Ethanol	Increased BP lowering	Vasodilation
Haloperidol	Decreased BP lowering	Antagonism

Table continued on following page

TABLE 7–1.   DRUG INTERACTIONS INVOLVING ANTIHYPERTENSIVE AGENTS (Continued)

Interacting Drugs	Adverse Effect	Probable Mechanism
Norepinephrine	Increased response to norepinephrine	Decreased uptake (reduced inactivation) of norepinephrine
MAO inhibitors	Decreased BP lowering	Uncertain
Hydralazine when mixed into glucose-containing IV fluids	Potential for formation of toxic hydrazones	Not defined?
Methyldopa with		
Haloperidol	Increased haloperidol toxicity	Uncertain
Tolbutamide	Increased hypoglycemia	Inhibition of hepatic microsomal enzymes
Lithium	Increased lithium toxicity	Uncertain
Tricyclic antidepressants	Decreased BP lowering	Inhibition of uptake of methyldopa at effector site?
Levodopa	Decreased levodopa effect	Not defined
Phenothiazines	Increased BP lowering	Inhibition of uptake of alpha-methyl norepinephrine at effector site?
Propranolol with		
Barbiturates	Decreased beta-blocker effect	Induction of hepatic microsomal enzymes
Chlorpromazine	Increased effects of both drugs	Inhibition of metabolism of both drugs
Insulin or oral hypoglycemics	Prolonged hypoglycemia	Decreased glycogenolysis
	Masking of tachycardia and tremor	Beta-receptor blockade
	Paradoxical hypertension and/or vasoconstriction during hypoglycemia	Unopposed alpha effect of epinephrine
Lidocaine	Increased lidocaine effect	Decreased lidocaine clearance
Theophylline	Increased theophylline effect	Decreased theophylline clearance
Nifedipine	Hypotension, congestive heart failure	Additive effect
Verapamil	Severe bradycardia	Additive effect

Potassium-sparing diuretics with		
Beta-blocker	Increased chance of hyperkalemia	Additional interference with potassium homeostasis
Nonsteroidal anti-inflammatory agents	Increased chance of hyperkalemia	As above
Potassium supplements	Increased chance of hyperkalemia	As above
Diuretics with		
Salicylates	Increased CNS toxicity with acetazolamide	Increased brain levels
Digitalis preparations	Increased digitalis toxicity	Hypokalemia
d-Tubocurarine	Increased curariform effect	Hypokalemia
Lithium	Increased lithium toxicity	Decreased lithium excretion
Corticosteroids such as predisone or cortisone	Increased hypokalemia	Additive effect
Reserpine with		
Digitalis preparations	Increased arrhythmic risk	Not established
Levodopa	Decreased levodopa effect	Not defined
Sympathomimetic amines with		
Tricyclic antidepressants	Hypertension, hypertensive crisis	Inhibition of norepinephrine uptake
MAO inhibitors	Severe hypertension	Increase in storage and release of norepinephrine
Indomethacin	Severe hypertension	Not defined
All antihypertensives	Decreased BP lowering	Antagonistic effect
MAO inhibitors with		
Levodopa	Hypertensive crisis, but not if taking carbidopa	Increase in storage and release of dopamine, norepinephrine, or both
Meperidine	Hypertension, hypotension, coma	Unknown
Hypoglycemics	Increased hypoglycemia	Not defined
Tricyclic antidepressants	Seizures, hyperpyrexia	Not defined

Habit-Food-Drug Interactions

Although most clinicians are aware of pharmacologic interactions that may influence antihypertensive therapy, they should also be cognizant of nondrug events that may aggravate hypertension and offset therapeutic intervention. Common examples include smoking and isometric exercise.

Food Interactions with Drugs. Patients taking MAO inhibitors who eat large amounts of tyramine-containing food or wine (aged cheeses, chianti) may develop severe hypertension. This is believed to be caused by the catecholamine-releasing property of tyramine.

Smoking Interactions with Drugs. It is well established that smoking alters the disposition and action of many drugs. Most of the known smoking-drug interactions involve cigarette smoking. Little is known about the effect of pipe or cigar smoking on drug action, but it is likely that interactions could occur with heavy use of pipes or cigars, especially if the smoke is inhaled.

These smoking-induced alterations appear to involve stimulation of hepatic metabolism of the drugs, resulting in a reduction of their levels in the blood. This enzyme induction is probably caused by the polycyclic hydrocarbons present in tobacco smoke. Drug metabolism appears to be stimulated predominantly in young and middle-aged smokers; older patients seem relatively resistant to this effect. Although enzyme induction is the primary mechanism of reported smoking-drug interactions, tobacco smoke contains other substances (e.g., nicotine) that may affect drug action.

Smoking has been associated with reduced serum propranolol levels and increased propranolol clearance in both patients and normal subjects receiving chronic oral doses of propranolol. Furthermore, at least two studies have shown that smoking inhibits the expected therapeutic effect of propranolol in the treatment of angina pectoris.

Smoking and propranolol have both been reported to affect the peripheral circulation adversely, so the combination should be viewed with caution in predisposed patients. It is not known whether smoking may increase propranolol dosage requirements, but one should be alert for the possibility. Smoking should be discouraged if the propranolol is being used for hypertension.

Finally, a caveat regarding the interaction of beta-blockers and smoking in general is in order. Although most studies have focused on the adverse effects of propranolol, a recent preliminary report suggests that the interaction of smoking with propranolol may not necessarily extend to all beta-blockers. For example, the attenuation of the antihypertensive response of propranolol by coffee and smoking does not appear to obtain for the cardioselective agent atenolol.

Isometric Exercise. The potential effects of isometric exercise upon the blood pressure and the cardiovascular system are not widely appreciated. Sustained isometric activity may markedly increase both heart rate and the systolic blood pressure, the latter at times reaching levels over 200 mm Hg, even in individuals without pre-existing hypertension. Examples of isometric activity include such mundane activities as carrying a heavy suitcase from one's car to the airport terminal. It should be emphasized that it is not merely the lifting of a heavy object, but the carrying of it as well that may be associated with marked and at times frightening elevations in blood pressure. One can envisage the potentially dangerous aspects of hemodynamic changes in a patient with a history of previous cerebral vascular accident.

REFERENCES

Hansten, PD: Drug Interactions, 4th ed. Lea & Febiger, Philadelphia, 1979.

MacLennan, WJ: Drug Interactions. Gerontol Clin 16:18–24, 1974.

Blaschke, TF, Cohen, SN, Tatro, DS, and Rubin, PC: Drug-drug interactions and aging. *In* Jarvik, LF, Greenblatt, DJ, and Harman, D (eds.): Clinical Pharmacology and the Aged Patient. Raven Press, New York, 1981, pp. 11–26.

Adverse interactions of drugs. Med Lett Drugs Ther 23(5):17–28, 1981.

Lloyd-Mostyn, RH, and Oram, S: Modification by propranolol of cardiovascular effects of induced hypoglycaemia. Lancet I:1213–1215, 1975.

McLaren, EH: Severe hypertension produced by interaction of phenylpropanolamine with methyldopa and oxprenolol. Br Med J 2:283–284, 1976.

Bailey, RR, and Neale, TJ: Rapid clonidine withdrawal with blood pressure overshoot exaggerated by beta-blockade. Br Med J 1:942–943, 1976.

Belz, GG, Doering, W, Munkes, R, and Matthews, J: Interaction between digoxin and calcium antagonists and antiarrhythmic drugs. Clin Pharmacol Ther 33:410–417, 1983.

Smoking interactions with drugs. Drug Interactions Newsletter 2(4):13–16, April 1982.

Furosemide and ibuprofen. Drug Interactions Newsletter 1(12):48–49, December 1981.

Calcium channel blocker interactions. Drug Interactions Newsletter 2(7):27–30, July 1982.

8

FACTORS IN THE CHOICE OF AN ANTIHYPERTENSIVE DRUG

Most physicians have a "favorite" antihypertensive medication, used perhaps because of the confidence that comes with familiarity. Aside from familiarity, however, how should a physician choose a medication(s) for a given patient? The principal factors that we use are listed in Table 8–1 and discussed below.

1. Antihypertensive Effects. Despite extravagant claims made by the proponents of varying classes of antihypertensive agents, it must be emphasized that, with a few possible exceptions, most of the available medications, when used appropriately, are approximately similar in their antihypertensive efficacy.

2. Safety. In light of the approximately equivalent antihypertensive efficacy and the wide spectrum of adverse effects that attend the use of the several classes of antihypertensive drugs, the clinician must consider side effects as a major factor when choosing an antihypertensive agent.

3. Patient Acceptance. Although certain adverse effects of drugs may not necessarily be a threat to the well-being of a patient, they may be sufficiently disturbing to interfere with drug acceptance and hence compliance. Examples

TABLE 8–1. FACTORS IN THE CHOICE OF AN ANTIHYPERTENSIVE DRUG

1. Antihypertensive effects
2. Safety
3. Patient acceptance
4. Cost
5. Number of doses per day
6. Need for laboratory follow-up
7. Mechanism of action
8. Potential interaction with other drugs
9. Additional salutary effects

include impotence with the use of guanethidine or somnolence and decreased mental activity noted commonly with administration of several of the sympatholytic agents.

4. **Cost.** All too frequently the physician prescribes a specific drug without bothering to determine if another agent within the same class and with similar properties may have a distinct cost advantage to the patient. It cannot be overemphasized that a considerable cost differential may exist for medications that might be interchangeable for a given patient (Table 8–2).

5. **Number of Doses Per Day.** Although compliance is by no means assured by a medication that can be taken once daily, most patients prefer the simplest regimen, and this is an important factor in the choice of a drug. Fortunately, several antihypertensive medications can now be taken either once a day (i.e., the diuretic chlorthalidone, the beta-blocker atenolol) or twice a day (numerous agents, including the sympatholytic drugs clonidine and guanabenz, several beta-blockers, and the vasodilator hydralazine).

6. **Need for Laboratory Follow-up.** An additional consideration that is often overlooked in choosing a medication is the need for laboratory follow-up. For example, in general, the metabolic complications associated with the use of diuretics are more extensive than those occurring with the sympatholy-

TABLE 8–2. RELATIVE COST OF ANTIHYPERTENSIVE AGENTS*

Drug	Dosage Regimen	Daily Cost	Cost/100
Hydrochlorothiazide (Esidrix)	50 mg daily	$0.08	$ 8.40
Chlorthalidone (Hygroton)	50 mg daily	0.17	17.10
Amiloride (Midamor)	5 mg daily	0.17	16.88
Spironolactone (Aldactone)	25 mg twice daily	0.44	21.80
Triamterene (50 mg) and hydrochlorothiazide (25 mg) (Dyazide)	one twice daily	0.26	26.20
Furosemide (Lasix)	40 mg daily	0.12	12.45
Ethacrynic acid (Edecrin)	50 mg daily	0.15	14.95
Metolazone (Zaroxolyn)	5 mg daily	0.15	14.96
Guanabenz (Wytensin)	4 mg twice daily	0.40	20.00
Methyldopa (Aldomet)	250 mg three times daily	0.44	14.86
Clonidine (Catapres)	0.1 mg twice daily	0.30	14.90
Reserpine	0.25 mg daily	0.014	1.42
Guanethidine (Ismelin)	10 mg daily	0.21	21.17
Prazosin (Minipres)	1 mg twice daily	0.28	13.38
Propranolol (Inderal)	40 mg twice daily	0.23	11.75
Atenolol (Tenormin)	50 mg daily	0.32	32.26
Nadolol (Corgard)	40 mg daily	0.32	32.63
Pindolol (Visken)	5 mg twice daily	0.28	14.40
Timolol (Blocadren)	10 mg twice daily	0.44	22.19
Hydralazine (Apresoline)	25 mg four times daily	0.36	8.98
Minoxidil (Loniten)	2.5 mg twice daily	0.32	16.31
Captopril (Capoten)	25 mg three times daily	0.75	25.00
Nifedipine (Procardia)	10 mg three times daily	0.62	20.78

*Prices represent average wholesale cost as detailed in *Drug Topics Redbook, 1983,* published by Medical Economics Co., Oradell, NJ.

TABLE 8–3. USE OF ANTIHYPERTENSIVE DRUGS IN PATIENTS WITH UNDERLYING PROBLEMS

Symptom or Condition	Drugs Tending to Mitigate the Problem	Drugs Tending to Exacerbate (or Confound) the Problem
Anxiety	Beta-blockers Reserpine Clonidine Methyldopa Guanabenz	Pargyline
Insomnia	Reserpine Clonidine Methyldopa Guanabenz	Beta-blockers Pargyline
Headache	Propranolol Reserpine Clonidine Methyldopa	Hydralazine Minoxidil Prazosin
Palpitations	Beta-blockers Reserpine Clonidine Methyldopa Guanabenz Calcium-entry blockers	Pargyline
Functional diarrhea	Clonidine Guanabenz	Reserpine Guanethidine
Diabetes		Diuretics Beta-blockers
Gout		Diuretics
Liver disease		Methyldopa

tics. For instance, hypokalemia is not a side-effect of inhibitors of the sympathetic nervous system.

Patients receiving diuretics, therefore, usually require more frequent laboratory determinations, at least during the first year of therapy. Such a consideration may influence patient acceptance and compliance, since the cost of required laboratory examinations may nullify, at least in part, the cost advantage of a certain class of drugs.

7. Mechanism of Action. The availability of numerous antihypertensive agents means that the clinician has access to medications that act by differing mechanisms. The physician can take advantage of these differences by selecting antihypertensive agents to meet a specific treatment goal. As an example, in a young patient with systolic hypertension related to a hyperadrenergic state, one might select a beta-blocker whose primary mode of action is to lower the heart rate and thus cardiac output.

8. Potential Interaction with Other Drugs. As discussed above, pharmacologic interactions are an important consideration in the selection of an antihypertensive agent, whether at Step-1 or when adding an additional agent. As an example, if a patient requires a tricyclic antidepressant, one should avoid the use of guanethidine, methyldopa, or clonidine as the antihypertensive agent.

9. Additional Salutary Effects. A final consideration in the selection of an antihypertensive drug is the additional salutary effects afforded by such agents.

For example, one may wish to select a beta-blocker as the initial antihypertensive drug in patients with myocardial infarction who may simultaneously benefit from the cardioprotective effects of these agents. Table 8–3 provides a compilation of antihypertensive agents that tend to either mitigate or exacerbate various underlying conditions.

FACTORS IN THE CHOICE OF A STEP-1 ANTIHYPERTENSIVE DRUG

Using the above broad guidelines, one can rationally approach the selection of a Step-1 drug. As noted, there is considerable controversy with regard to what the appropriate Step-1 antihypertensive agent should be. Currently, there are no large-scale, definitive data to document a substantial advantage in either efficacy or patient accceptance of any specific type of drug therapy. Two such trials are now underway, however, both comparing a diuretic with a beta-blocking drug. One study involves 5000 Swedish men (Wilhelmsen et al., 1981), and the other includes 18,000 English patients (Medical Research Council Working Party, 1981). It will likely be another two to five years before the results of these two trials are available. Although there is no consensus regarding this issue, we would like to review those specific factors that should be considered by the clinician. Table 8–4 summarizes those factors that must be weighed in any such decision.

1. Although agents other than diuretics and beta-blockers have been proposed as Step-1 drugs, at the present time the overwhelming majority of physicians believe that either diuretics or beta-blockers should be selected as the Step-1 agent.
2. Initial suggestions for the superiority of beta-blockers over diuretics have not been substantiated, and it is now clear that, in general, both classes of drugs are equally efficacious in their antihypertensive effects.
3. Both beta-blockers and diuretics produce symptomatic side effects. Although not inordinate with either class of agent, side effects are probably

TABLE 8–4. FACTORS INFLUENCING THE CHOICE OF DIURETICS VS. BETA-BLOCKERS AS STEP-1 AGENTS

In Favor of Diuretics	In Favor of Beta-Blockers
Less expensive	A young patient with systolic hypertension
Fewer side effects (e.g., less fatigue, no insomnia)	Another indication for beta-blockers, such as recent myocardial infarction or migraine headaches
Less-serious side effects (e.g., congestive heart failure is not produced)	Perhaps somewhat greater potency in certain patients
Fewer absolute or relative contraindications (e.g., congestive heart failure, heart block, marked peripheral vascular disease, bronchospasm are not contraindications)	When diuretic-induced hypokalemia is a problem
Fewer drug interactions	Somewhat lesser need for laboratory surveillance (e.g., hypokalemia is not produced)
An older patient (over 60 years)	A patient with gout
In general, a simpler regimen and titration procedure	
Greater long-term experience	

more commonly noted with beta-blockers. Initial claims for the superiority of beta-blockers entailed a lessened frequency of biochemical side effects with these agents. Earlier claims that beta-blockers induced substantially fewer biochemical side effects have not been borne out. For example, although hypokalemia is not seen with beta-blockers, these agents tend to produce abnormalities of lipid and carbohydrate metabolism similar to those observed with diuretic administration.

4. Patient acceptance is good for both of these classes of agents; nevertheless, it appears that, because of side effects such as insomnia, nightmares, headaches, and dizziness, the drop-out rate is somewhat higher with beta-blockers.

5. Largely because of the need to periodically check serum potassium, the requirement for periodic laboratory testing is greater with patients taking diuretics than with those taking beta-blockers. In light of the known propensity for diuretics to induce diverse metabolic and electrolyte abnormalities (see Chapter 6) serum electrolytes, uric acid, BUN, and creatinine should be determined periodically. In reality, a single automated determination is probably as cost effective as ordering fewer of these tests individually. Beta-blocker therapy mandates periodic tests as well. In this case, a chest x-ray to assess for increasing cardiomegaly and an ECG suffice. With both classes of agents, plasma lipid evaluations should be carried out both before and during therapy, since either type of medication may alter blood lipids in an unfavorable direction.

6. Both diuretic agents and certain beta-blockers can be prescribed once a day in order to reduce blood pressure. In this regard, it should be emphasized that the available data indicate that most beta-blockers must be taken at least twice a day to obtain their cardioprotective effects.

7. Another consideration, which has received extensive publicity, is the cardioprotective effects of the beta-blocker agents. It is clear that beta-blockers reduce the risk of second myocardial infarction and sudden death in a patient with a recent myocardial infarction. It should be remembered, however, that there are no data available *at present* demonstrating a primary protective effect (i.e., against an initial myocardial infarction).

8. Finally, a major consideration differentiating the two classes of agents is cost. In most Western countries today, beta-blockers are several times more expensive than the usual doses of diuretics necessary to lower blood pressure to a similar degree.

Having weighed factors that enter into a decision for prescribing a Step-1 drug, it is apparent that one can prescribe either a diuretic or a beta-blocker in the majority of essential hypertensive patients. We believe that diuretics should be used with greater caution in patients with overt diabetes or gout. On the other hand, beta-blockers should not be used in patients with atrial-ventricular conduction defects and obstructive lung disease. After excluding the above contraindications, one is left with approximately 75 per cent of the essential hypertensive population who are amenable to either mode of therapy. Our own recommendation is to favor the use of beta-blockers in the young patient, especially if he has systolic hypertension and does not engage in vigorous physical exercise. We recommend diuretics as the Step-1 drug in patients above the age of 55 and perhaps in black patients. Furthermore, one may lean toward the use of a beta-blocker in patients with a history of a recent myocardial infarction.

TABLE 8–5. ANTIHYPERTENSIVE AGENTS WHOSE USE FOR MONOTHERAPY HAS BEEN SUGGESTED

1. Beta-blockers
2. Clonidine
3. Methyldopa
4. Captopril
5. Prazosin
6. Guanabenz
7. Nifedipine

NONDIURETIC MONOTHERAPY FOR HYPERTENSION

Nondiuretic monotherapy is a relatively new and controversial topic in the field of antihypertensive management. For the purpose of this discussion we define *monotherapy* as the use of a single agent, other than a diuretic, for the therapy of hypertension. Of course, during premarketing trials, every antihypertensive agent must have been shown to lower the blood pressure to a greater degree than a placebo. This does not imply, however, that the medication is suitable for long-term monotherapy. For example, when hydralazine is employed by itself, the antihypertensive efficacy is short lived because of the blood pressure–elevating influences of increases in cardiac output and fluid retention. Of interest, limited preliminary evidence suggests that sodium retention is not a concomitant of chronic monotherapy with clonidine or guanabenz.

A list of several of the medications that have been suggested for this approach is shown in Table 8–5. Because monotherapy has been already discussed with respect to beta-blockers (regarding the question of diuretics versus beta-blockers), we will not include that specific aspect herein. One reason for the controversy attending the subject of nondiuretic monotherapy is the meagerness of specific data in the literature (except regarding beta-blockers). Our discussion, therefore, will be in general terms.

The potential advantages of monotherapy are shown in Table 8–6. They include simplicity, fewer metabolic side effects (in comparison to diuretics), provision of additional therapeutic benefits (such as relief of angina), and perhaps, in some cases, greater potency. On the other hand, there are several potential disadvantages (Table 8–7), which include the above-mentioned possibility of tolerance or pseudotolerance, greater incidence of postural or exercise-induced hypotension, the more complicated titration process, and the risk of a

TABLE 8–6. PURPORTED DESIRABLE FEATURES OF MONOTHERAPY FOR HYPERTENSION

1. Simplicity
2. Increased potency
3. Fewer metabolic side effects
4. Improved compliance
5. Ease of adding additional agents if necessary, particularly a diuretic
6. Additional therapeutic benefits, such as relief of angina

TABLE 8–7. POTENTIAL DISADVANTAGES OF MONOTHERAPY FOR HYPERTENSION

1. Step-Care (diuretic first) is still the "official line"
2. Loss of additive effect of multiple agents
3. Limited number of proven appropriate agents
4. Insufficient potency for many patients, even those with mild hypertension
5. Some agents are relatively expensive
6. Some agents require multiple doses
7. Loss of counterbalancing of certain side effects
8. Possibility of tolerance or pseudotolerance
9. Greater incidence of postural or exercise-induced hypotension
10. Need for higher dose of agents, which increases the time for titration, the chance of side effects, and the cost
11. Withdrawal syndromes may be more problematic than with diuretics
12. More of a problem if unexpected surgery is necessary

withdrawal syndrome. Additionally, two very important disadvantages are a markedly greater cost to the patient and the fact that for complete blood pressure control relatively large doses will often be required, even in patients with mild hypertension. Unfortunately, this latter consideration augments not only the cost but the chance of undesirable, even limiting side effects (see case examples 10 and 14).

At this juncture, what should be the viewpoint of the clinician, who may be bombarded with promotional material regarding the value of monotherapy with this or that antihypertensive medication? We recommend an open-minded approach, because nondiuretic monotherapy may prove to be excellent therapy in many patients. As we have emphasized, this often appears to be the case with beta-blockers. Furthermore, if a patient is begun on monotherapy with inadequate control of the blood pressure, a diuretic can certainly be added easily enough, with a final result not necessarily much different from that of starting with the diuretic first. On the other hand, except for a limited number of selected patients, we believe that much more information is needed before nondiuretic monotherapy (other than with beta-blockers) can be recommended for widespread application.

REFERENCES

Editorial: Antihypertensive drugs, plasma lipids, and coronary disease. Lancet II:19–20, 1980.

Wilhelmsen, L, Berglund, G, Elmfeldt, D, and Wedel, H: Beta-blockers versus saluretics in hypertension. Prev Med 10:38–49, 1981.

Medical Research Council Working Party. Adverse reactions to bendroflumethiazide and propranolol for the treatment of mild hypertension. Lancet II:539–542, 1981.

Nondiuretic Monotherapy

Campese, VM, Romoff, M, Telfer, N, Weidmann, P, and Massry, SG: Role of sympathetic nerve inhibition and body sodium-volume state in the antihypertensive action of clonidine in essential hypertension. Kidney Int 18:351–357, 1980.

Walker, BR, Deitch, MW, Schneider, BE, Hare, LE, and Gold, JA: Long-term therapy of hypertension with guanabenz. Clin Ther 47:217–228, 1981.

Thananopavarn, C, Golub, MS, Eggena, P, Barrett, JD, and Sambhi, MP: Clonidine, a centrally acting sympathetic inhibitor as monotherapy for mild to moderate hypertension. Am J Cardiol 49:153–158, 1982.

Kaplan, NM (guest ed.): Proceedings of a symposium: Initial therapy in hypertension. Am J Cardiol 51:619–660, 1983.

9

DISCONTINUATION SYNDROME AND STEP-DOWN THERAPY

Discontinuation Syndrome (DS)

The spectrum of adverse clinical events following the abrupt cessation of any pharmacologic agent has been termed the discontinuation syndrome. Although interest in this problem has centered on antihypertensive agents in general, and the sympatholytic medication clonidine in particular, it is clear that the DS may occur not only after the abrupt discontinuation of many antihypertensive drugs (Table 9–1), but after discontinuation of many other medications as well, including the benzodiazepines. The typical clinical signs and symptoms (Table 9–2) are those of enhanced sympathetic activity, angina (with beta-blockers), and acute elevations in blood pressure, with its possible adverse effects. Although worrisome hypertension need not be a component of the syndrome, the blood pressure may rapidly return to pretreatment levels as the drug effect dissipates. Such a rise may be either asymptomatic or associated with potentially severe complications. Rarely, so-called overshoot

TABLE 9–1. ANTIHYPERTENSIVE DRUGS THAT HAVE PRODUCED DISCONTINUATION SYNDROME

1. Centrally acting drugs
   a. Clonidine
   b. Methyldopa
2. Beta-adrenoreceptor–blocking agents
3. Other antihypertensive drugs
   a. Guanethidine
   b. Reserpine
4. Combination therapy
   a. Centrally acting drugs and beta-blockers
   b. Centrally acting drugs and diuretics
   c. Beta-blockers and diuretics

TABLE 9–2.   CLINICAL SIGNS AND SYMPTOMS ASSOCIATED WITH THE DISCONTINUATION SYNDROME

1. Signs and symptoms related to enhanced sympathetic activity
   a. Nervousness and restlessness
   b. Palpitations
   c. Abdominal discomfort
   d. Headache
   e. Tremor
   f. Diaphoresis
   g. Tachycardia
   h. Angina or myocardial infarction in predisposed patients (predominantly after withdrawal of beta-blocker)
2. Signs and symptoms related to rebound or overshoot hypertension
   a. Any type of hypertensive crisis such as hypertensive encephalopathy
   b. Acute myocardial infarction
   c. Sudden death

hypertension may occur, which means a rapid rise of blood pressure to a level in excess of the pretreatment status.

The pathophysiologic mechanisms of this discontinuation syndrome are uncertain and controversial. For the centrally acting drugs, they probably relate, at least in part, to increased levels of circulating catecholamines, increased sensitivity of adrenergic receptors to circulating catecholamines, or both factors. It seems likely that the increase in the number of beta-adrenergic receptors that attends the long-term administration of beta-blockers plays an important role with these agents. Indeed, ISA-positive members of the group, which possibly do not increase receptor density, appear to have a diminished risk of inducing the DS. The factors believed to predispose patients to the DS are shown in Table 9–3. Perhaps most important is the sudden termination of high doses of a centrally acting antiadrenergic agent or of combination therapy. There is good evidence that the risk of DS is enhanced by discontinuation of clonidine in a patient who continues to ingest a beta-adrenergic inhibitor. Knowledge of these factors is important because it permits a greater opportunity for prevention. A gradual tapering of medication over 7 to 10 days will usually obviate the DS. Treatment of DS revolves around the reinitiated use of the offending drug and, if necessary, hospitalization, bed rest, and administration of a parenteral agent such as nitroprusside or, if appropriate, phentolamine.

TABLE 9–3   POSSIBLE FACTORS PREDISPOSING PATIENTS TO DISCONTINUATION SYNDROME

1. Abrupt discontinuation of antihypertensive drug therapy
2. Centrally acting drugs and beta-blockers
3. Combination drug therapy—especially centrally acting drugs with beta-blockers
4. High daily doses of antihypertensive drug
5. Severely elevated pretreatment blood pressure
6. Renin status—high or normal renin hypertension
7. Renovascular hypertension or renal disease
8. Postoperative state
9. Ischemic heart disease

Step-Down Therapy

An often-asked question is what to do with a patient whose blood pressure has been controlled by pharmacologic means for several months or longer. Specifically, should the dosage of some or all of the agents be tapered? Should the number of drugs in a multiple-drug regimen be reduced? As is the case in other areas of hypertension, this is a controversial subject. There is some evidence suggesting that chronic control of the blood pressure is associated with alteration of baroreceptor function or other unknown mechanisms that may permit a reduction of antihypertensive dosage in some patients. At the present time, our recommendation is that after a minimum of a year of good blood pressure control (i.e., diastolic blood pressure of 85 mm Hg or less), the physician may elect to reduce gradually the dosage of medications, one agent at a time. Probably, in most patients, this will be associated after a variable delay with a gradual elevation in blood pressure. Some patients, however, will do well on a reduced dosage, fewer medications, or both. Obviously, if step-down is used, it is mandatory that the clinician follow the patient closely and that the patient not be lost to follow-up.

REFERENCES

Houston, MC: Abrupt cessation of treatment in hypertension: Consideration of clinical features, mechanisms, prevention and management of the discontinuation syndrome. Am Heart J 102:415–430, 1981.

Hart, GR, and Anderson, RJ: Withdrawal syndromes and cessation of antihypertensive therapy. Arch Intern Med. 141:1125–1127, 1981.

Levinson, PD, Khatri, IM, and Freis ED: Persistence of normal blood pressure after withdrawal of drug treatment in mild hypertension. Arch Intern Med 142:2265–2268, 1982.

McFate-Smith, W: Resetting of barostats revisited. Arch Intern Med 142:2263–2264, 1982.

III

Treatment of Specific Types of Hypertension

10

MILD HYPERTENSION

Mild hypertension (Table 10–1) may be defined by diastolic blood pressures (DBP's) between 90 and 99 mm Hg (and/or systolic pressures between 140 and 160 mm Hg). Whether to treat mild hypertension has become a topic of considerable controversy. The question is of more than academic interest, since at least 40 million persons in the United States have pressures in this range, and it has been conservatively estimated that the yearly cost of treating this number of patients might be $20 billion. Although it is now almost universally accepted that for patients with DBP greater than 100 mm Hg the potential risks of medical therapy are far outweighed by the benefits, the value vs. risk conundrum remains unresolved in patients with mild hypertension, despite the recent publication of the data from several large multicenter trials.

Although the results of the American Hypertension Detection and Follow-up Program (HDFP) study have been widely quoted as providing clear-cut evidence for the value of therapy for mild hypertension, several editorial comments on the subject have criticized the design of the study. For example, Dr. Edward Freis, who designed most of the Veterans Administration Cooperative Studies on antihypertensive agents, drew the following conclusions in a recent review:

1. Evidence supporting the value of medical treatment of borderline and mild hypertension is not clearly established.

2. Interpretation of the most favorable results (HDFP) is confounded because of study design.

3. The better conducted studies on mild hypertension reported either fluctuating results or no indication of benefit.

4. Two smaller, earlier, controlled trials (Veterans Administration and U.S. Public Health Service) found no significant benefit of treatment in mild or borderline hypertension.

In agreement with the opinion of Dr. Freis, at the present time we propose the following recommendations for the patient with a diastolic blood pressure between 90 and 99 mm Hg.

1. Remember that blood pressure may fall without drug treatment in many patients.

2. Because of the possibility of benefit, even though unproved, a compromise position may be most appropriate.

TABLE 10–1. MILD HYPERTENSION

1. Defined as diastolic blood pressure between 90 and 99 mm Hg, systolic pressure between 140 and 160 mm Hg
2. Does patient have "office" hypertension?
3. Carries increased risk of cardiovascular morbidity, and may progress to moderate-to-severe hypertension
4. Look for excessive use of salt, or use of vasopressors such as nasal sprays, cold remedies, or oral contraceptives
5. Therapy appears to reduce morbidity, but the issue remains controversial
6. Modified Step-Care approach is valid, but choice of medications is not established

The patient with few or no other coronary artery disease (CAD) risk factors should be placed on a weight-reducing program, a low-sodium diet without drugs, or both, and followed periodically to detect progression to more severe hypertension. Contrariwise, patients with many CAD risk factors may have their blood pressure reduced with drugs, using the Step-Care approach and avoiding complicated, multiple-drug regimens and excessive decrements in blood pressure.

Recently, the World Health Organization (WHO) has recommended a specific and practical guideline for the management of a patient whose blood pressure is between 90 and 105 mm Hg. This approach is summarized in algorithmic form in Figure 10–1.

According to this method, when a patient is observed to have a diastolic blood pressure above 90 mm Hg, the measurement should be repeated on at least two occasions over the subsequent four weeks. This permits appropriate reassessment, because, as mentioned earlier in the book, in a large proportion of patients both systolic and diastolic pressures decrease if the observations are repeated over a period of time.

If the diastolic pressure is found after four weeks to have fallen below 100 mm Hg, drug treatment is not instituted, but further observations are made over the next three months. Subsequently, if diastolic pressure increases, or in patients in whom it remained persistently above 100 mm Hg during the initial four-week period, antihypertensive treatment should be commenced.

After three months, treatment should be begun if the diastolic pressure continues to exceed 95 mm Hg. If the pressure is less than 95 mm Hg, the patient is then followed at six-month intervals. Some patients whose diastolic pressure remains in the range of 90 to 94 mm Hg are exposed to an increased risk of vascular disease; if they are not treated, they should continue to be monitored at intervals of about three months. If at any subsequent examination the diastolic pressure exceeds 95 mm Hg and remains above this level on repeated examinations, drug treatment should be commenced.

The WHO allows that factors other than diastolic blood pressure frequently influence the decision to begin therapy. These include:

1. Systolic hypertension, an additional risk factor at any given level of diastolic pressure, favors treatment.

2. A strong family history of stroke or heart disease militates for a decision to treat.

3. *Age:* It has not been proven that patients over the age of 70 necessarily benefit from therapy, but it has been suggested that such patients *who are in good health* should not be differentiated from younger individuals. Con-

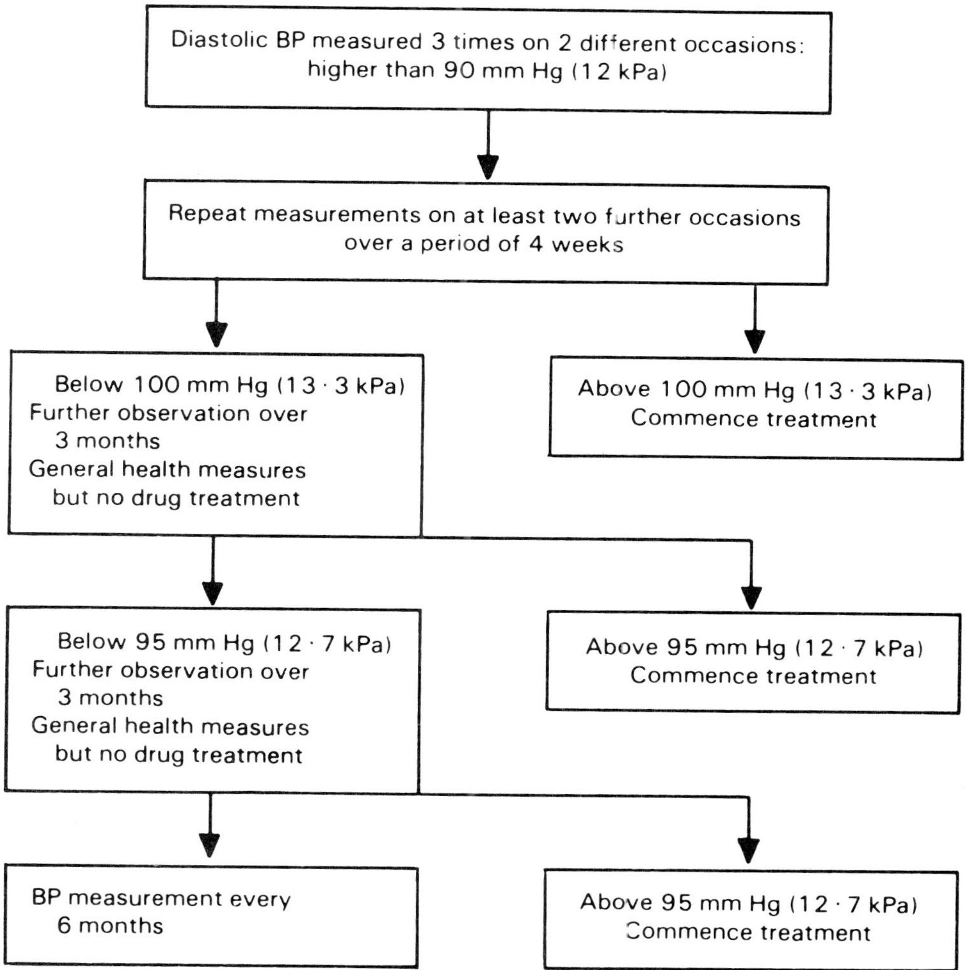

Definition and management of mild hypertension.

FIGURE 10–1. An algorithmic approach to the management of the patient with mild hypertension. According to this method, when a patient is observed to have a diastolic blood pressure above 90 mm Hg, the measurement should be repeated on at least two occasions over the subsequent four weeks. This permits appropriate reassessment, because, as mentioned earlier in the book, in a large proportion of patients both systolic and diastolic pressures decrease if the observations are repeated over a period of time. If the diastolic pressure is found after four weeks to have fallen below 100 mm Hg, drug treatment is not instituted, but further observations are made over the next three months. Subsequently, if diastolic pressure increases, or in patients in whom it remained persistently above 100 mm Hg during the initial four-week period, antihypertensive treatment should be commenced. After three months, treatment should be begun if the diastolic pressure continues to exceed 95 mm Hg. If the pressure is less than 95 mm Hg, the patient is then followed at six month intervals. Some patients whose diastolic pressure remains in the range of 90 to 94 mm Hg are exposed to an increased risk of vascular disease; if they are not treated, they should continue to be monitored at intervals of about three months. If at any subsequent examination the diastolic pressure exceeds 95 mm Hg and remains above this level on repeated examinations, drug treatment should be commenced. (Reproduced with permission from Lancet I:457–458, 1983. Originally published in Bull WHO *61*(1):53–56, 1983.)

versely, patients with debilitating illnesses should not be given antihypertensive drug therapy unless their diastolic pressure consistently exceeds 105 mm Hg. Exceptions include elderly hypertensive patients with clear-cut cardiac failure who benefit from pharmacologic treatment, even if given for a short period of time.

4. Evidence of end-organ damage
   a. Left ventricular hypertrophy—as evidenced by clinical, radiologic, echocardiographic, or ECG criteria—warrants treatment.
   b. Retinal hemorrhages and exudates, although very rare in patients with mild hypertension, demand the prompt initiation of pharmacologic therapy.
   c. Unexplained proteinuria indicates possible renal damage and justifies therapy.

5. Coincident potentially fatal disease obviously influences management decisions.

REFERENCES

Hypertension Detection and Follow-up Program Cooperative Group: Five-year findings of the hypertension detection and follow-up program. Parts I and II. JAMA 242:2562–2577, 1979.

Report by the Management Committee: The Australian therapeutic trial in mild hypertension. Lancet I:1261–1267, 1980.

Editorial: The HDFP, the JNC, and nonpharmacologic management of hypertension. Mayo Clin Proc 55:651–652, 1980.

Helgeland, A: Treatment of mild hypertension: A five year controlled drug trial. The Oslo study. Am J Med 69:725–732, 1980.

Alderman, MH: Mild hypertension: New light on an old clinical controversy. Am J Med 69:653–655, 1980.

Moser, M: On the management of "mild hypertension." Arch Intern Med 141:1587–1588, 1981.

Madhavan, S, and Alderman, MH: The potential effect of blood pressure reduction on cardiovascular disease. A cautionary note. Arch Intern Med 141:1583–1586, 1981.

Multiple Risk Factor Intervention Trial Research Group: Multiple risk factor intervention trial. Risk factor changes and mortality results. JAMA 248:1465–1477, 1982.

Freis, ED: Should mild hypertension be treated? N Engl J Med 306:305–309, 1982.

Guidelines for the treatment of mild hypertension: memorandum from a WHO/ISH meeting. Lancet I:457–458, 1983.

Kaplan, NM (guest ed.): Proceedings of a symposium: Initial therapy in hypertension. Am J Cardiol 51:619–660, 1983.

11

ISOLATED SYSTOLIC HYPERTENSION AND HYPERTENSION IN THE ELDERLY

Two related nettlesome entities that the physician often encounters are isolated systolic hypertension and hypertension in the elderly (Tables 11–1 and 11–2). The latter topic was discussed recently in an excellent review by Hall and Wollam. Systolic hypertension is subdivided into two types: *isolated*, or pure, systolic hypertension and *disproportionate*, or dominant, systolic hypertension. In the former, the systolic blood pressure (SBP) is elevated but the diastolic blood pressure (DBP) is normal (i.e., SBP greater than or equal to 150 to 165 mm Hg and DBP less than 90 to 95 mm Hg). Disproportionate systolic hypertension is defined by a systolic blood pressure exceeding twice the figure obtained by subtracting 15 mm Hg from the diastolic pressure.

The data obtained by the National Health Examination Survey (1960–1962) were impressive in terms of the apparent frequency of systolic hypertension. Whereas, as expected, the frequency was extremely low below age 44, it occurred in 15 to 43 per cent of those above the age of 65. Disproportionate systolic hypertension is even more common. Furthermore, the Framingham Study demonstrated that isolated systolic hypertension carries a risk of cardiovascular morbidity that does not differ from that attributable to diastolic hypertension.

Although systolic blood pressure is influenced by the velocity of left ventricular ejection and the size of the stroke volume, the major determinant is the degree of aortic distensibility. Aortic inelasticity or rigidity increases with

TABLE 11–1. ISOLATED SYSTOLIC HYPERTENSION

1. More common in the elderly
2. Possibility of pseudohypertension should be considered
3. Risk of cardiovascular morbidity similar to that for diastolic hypertension
4. In general, treatment is more difficult than for combined systolic-diastolic hypertension
5. Value vs. risk of aggressive therapy not well established; side effects should be anticipated
6. Therapy must be individualized, and the goal should not be to reduce the systolic pressure to normal

TABLE 11–2. PRINCIPLES OF THERAPY OF HYPERTENSION IN THE ELDERLY

1. Consider possibility of pseudohypertension
2. Predominance of systolic hypertension is common
3. Therapeutic goals usually are not as great as in younger patients
4. Carefully assess patient for risks of undue hypotension such as cerebrovascular insufficiency
5. Follow patient carefully and frequently, especially at initiation of therapy or at time of changes in regimen
6. Watch closely for adverse effects of therapy, i.e., hypotension, postural hypotension, decreased perfusion of a vital organ, etc.
7. Use smaller than usual doses of medications, and increase dosages by small increments at infrequent intervals
8. Initiate therapy with small dose of diuretic (approximately one-half of usual dose)
    a. If blood pressure not controlled, increase diuretic dosage to usual level
    b. Subsequent choice of therapy is controversial, i.e., either hydralazine or clonidine, or methyldopa at low initial doses
    c. Although it has been suggested that beta-blockers may not be as effective in older as in younger patients and may cause more side effects in the former, this remains controversial
    d. Avoid agents or dosages tending to produce excessive sedation or change in mental status

age, and this is the major pathophysiologic abnormality accounting for the prevalence of systolic hypertension in the elderly. As mentioned above, a similar process in smaller arteries (brachial) accounts for the phenomenon of pseudohypertension, which should be suspected if a patient has very high levels of pressure without evidence of end-organ damage.

The mechanism of systolic hypertension in young patients is much less well understood. Preliminary data, however, suggest that increased ventricular ejection velocity, perhaps related to overactivity of the sympathetic nervous system, contributes importantly to the abnormality. Nevertheless, there is also evidence indicating that increased aortic rigidity may play a role even in young patients.

Hypertension in the Older Patient

As can be seen in Figure 11–1, increasing age is associated with a progressive increase in both systolic and diastolic blood pressure in men and women. Managing the older patient often presents the physician with a series of challenges. Currently, it is appreciated that much effort and determination are needed to make sure that elderly patients are neither deprived of effective treatment nor exposed to unnecessary risks. Benefits to heart and kidney aside, it is commonly felt that the primary consideration should be preventing stroke.

During sleep, when many strokes occur, cardiac output falls and considerable fluctuations in cerebral perfusion may occur. New standards must therefore be considered for all active antihypertensive treatments, especially because hypertension in the elderly is often characterized by higher systolic but lower diastolic pressure. When compared with younger groups, elderly patients have a lower cardiac output, impaired myocardial reserve, lesser aortic elasticity, higher total peripheral resistance, more contracted intravascular volume, and higher circulating norepinephrine levels.

Pharmacokinetic Changes in Aging

Several factors may complicate the response of elderly patients to antihypertensive agents. Both the selection and dosage of medications may need to be modified for the following reasons:

1. Impaired gastrointestinal absorption
2. Alteration of drug distribution related to loss of weight, reduction of total body water, and increased percentage of body fat
3. Changes in hepatic metabolism and renal excretion
4. Changes in protein binding

Lower body weight results in an increased dose of any medication per unit of weight, and therefore, the usual dose may have to be reduced. A given amount of water-soluble drug may have a smaller distribution and produce a higher blood level. Finally, fat-soluble drugs may have a greater distribution, resulting in lower blood levels. One of the major effects of these differences is to render elderly patients more susceptible to displacement interactions. For a more detailed consideration of this important topic, the reader is referred to recent publications by Vestal and Reidenberg.

Alterations in receptor "sensitivity" may exacerbate the problems of pharmacologic management. For some time, alterations in receptor sensitivity have been postulated to exist in elderly patients. Recent data obtained for propranolol indicate that there is an apparent decrease in sensitivity to beta-blockers in elderly patients. Finally, one of the most crucial yet least appreciated factors influencing drug response in the elderly is the impairment of biologic control systems. As an example, the fall in blood pressure produced by a combination

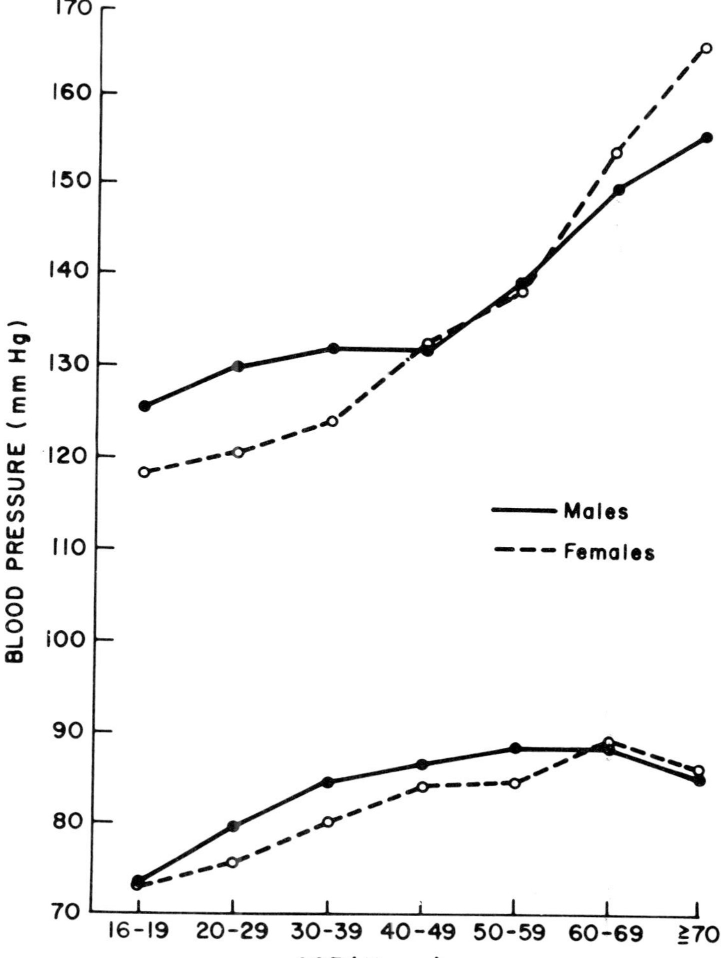

FIGURE 11–1. The effect of age on blood pressure. As can be seen, there is a progressive increase with age in both systolic and diastolic blood pressure in men and women. This phenomenon has been consistently noted in industrialized societies. (Reproduced by permission of the American Heart Association, Inc., from Kotchen, JM, et al.: Blood pressure trends with aging. Hypertension 4 [Suppl. III]:129, 1982.)

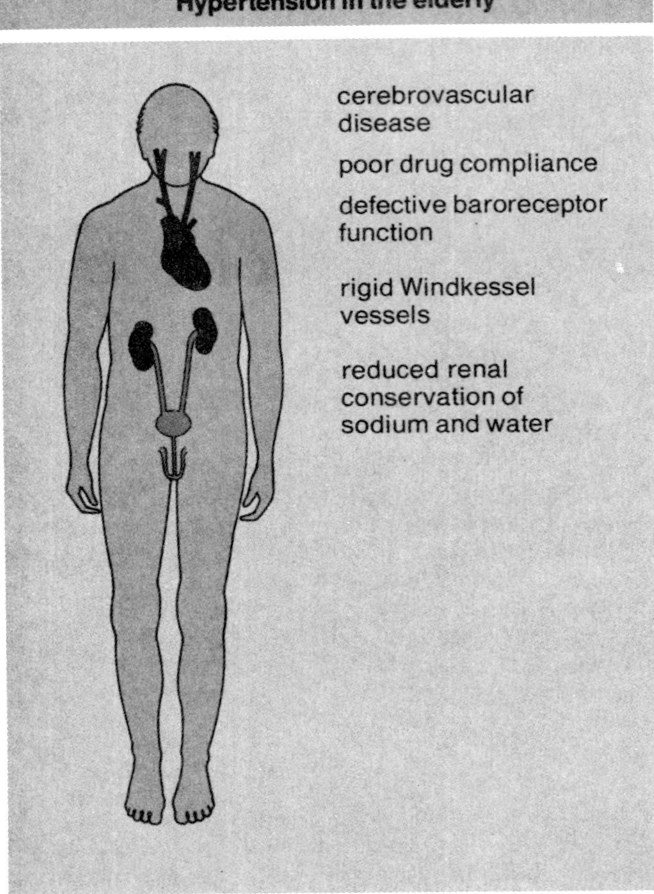

FIGURE 11–2. Features complicating the treatment of the elderly patient with hypertension. Because of the effects of several interrelated factors attributable to both the progression of hypertension per se and senescence, the elderly patient is subject to an increased risk of hypotension and its consequences. In addition, the reduced motivation and forgetfulness of the older patient exaggerates the commonly encountered problem of poor drug compliance. (Reproduced from Hypertension Illustrated by WS Peart, PS Sever, JD Swales, and R Tarazi, courtesy of Gower Medical Publishing.)

of hypotensive agents is likely to be much less effectively compensated for in elderly than in young patients. The relative inadequacy of homeostatic responses in older patients greatly enhances the likelihood that a greater than anticipated reduction in blood pressure will assume clinical importance.

Figure 11–2 schematically summarizes some of the peculiar clinical features of hypertension in the elderly patient. Unfortunately, these abnormalities, which include a tendency toward cerebral vascular insufficiency, rigid arteries, and defective baroreceptor function, acting in concert greatly enhance the risk of adverse ischemic complications of intervention with antihypertensive drugs. Poor drug compliance compounds the difficulties.

Treatment

There is evidence that in young patients with systolic hypertension, beta-blockers may be the agents of choice. On the other hand, the appropriate therapeutic approach to the management of isolated or predominant systolic hypertension in the elderly has not been established, and the topic is highly controversial. The value of therapy versus the risk of aggressive therapy is unknown.

All antihypertensives reduce both diastolic and systolic blood pressure. Except for direct vasodilators and prazosin, antihypertensives generally lower systolic pressures to a greater extent than diastolic. Thus, to reduce isolated systolic hypertension to normal may result in diastolic hypotension, the significance of which is unknown. Moreover the optimal level to which systolic blood pressure should be reduced has not been established. Levels of 140 mm Hg or less may be poorly tolerated by older patients. This may relate to the disordered autoregulation characteristic of chronic hypertension, that is, to the need of a mean arterial pressure greater than 110 mm Hg for adequate regulation of cerebral blood flow.

Not surprisingly, the treatment of elderly patients with systolic hypertension (and diastolic hypertension as well) appears to be associated with a higher incidence of hypotensive and ischemic complications than obtains with the therapy of younger subjects. This risk has been demonstrated not only with the potent agent guanethidine, but also with methyldopa, hydralazine, and low-dose minoxidil. Furthermore, the sensitivity to diuretics may be greatly increased. The reason for these problems has not been elucidated, but it may relate at least in part to a diminished response of plasma renin activity (PRA) and plasma aldosterone to sodium depletion, reduced sensitivity of the baroreceptor reflex mechanism, and impaired cerebral autoregulation.

In elderly patients with systolic hypertension, diuretics and other antihypertensives should be used in lower than usual doses and titrated slowly. In the absence of edema, loop-type diuretics should be avoided, and symptoms of potassium depletion, particularly ventricular ectopy, watched for carefully. Older patients appear to develop less tachycardia with the use of hydralazine, which seems to be efficacious in lowering the systolic blood pressure, but the risk of angina is substantial. We agree with the recommendation that therapy with hydralazine be initiated with very low doses (10 to 25 mg twice daily) and that in general it be combined with a low dose of a sympatholytic drug, which will limit any increase in cardiac work.

If beta-blockers are employed in elderly patients, one should watch closely for evidence of toxicity and begin with low doses, since there is some evidence that, for certain beta-blockers at least, the blood level of these medications tends to be higher and more variable in older patients. Furthermore, although inconclusive, there is a body of evidence indicating that, in general, beta-blockers may be less efficacious in older patients, and in older patients there are theoretic disadvantages to the use of agents such as beta-blockers that act by reducing cardiac output. Theoretically at least, beta-blockers with intrinsic sympathomimetic activity (ISA) might be preferable in the elderly, since they tend to control peaks of systolic blood pressure (which may be dangerous for elderly hypertensives), while tending to maintain the hemodynamic level needed for the aging hypertensive patient.

It has been suggested that centrally acting sympatholytic compounds, including methyldopa, clonidine, and guanabenz, may be appropriate medications for elderly hypertensive patients because they tend to preserve cardiac output and thus organ perfusion. At this time, however, the data are insufficient to allow a conclusive opinion. One should also remember that either alpha-receptor blockade or adrenergic neuron inhibition may cause postural problems.

Although there are a number of theoretic reasons to suspect that clinically significant drug interactions may occur with greater frequency in aging patients, there are virtually no data about the magnitude of the problem in this large and important segment of our population. Nevertheless, there is a general clinical impression that drug interactions are more common and lead to more adverse consequences in the aged than in younger patients.

Finally, it must be remembered that the problem of noncompliance, which is common in all patients, is often exaggerated in the elderly, in part because of forgetfulness and reduced motivation.

In summary, since the pertinent data are not available, we favor an approach to the treatment of elderly patients with hypertension not very dissimilar to that of the classic Step-Care method (with the above-mentioned caveats regarding very cautious titration). Thus, we recommend beginning therapy with diuretics and, if insufficient, adding very small doses of a sympatholytic agent. The patient must be seen at frequent intervals and the regimen changed appropriately at the first indication of an important adverse reaction.

REFERENCES

Systolic Hypertension

Kannel WB, Dawber, TR, and McGee, DL: Perspectives on systolic hypertension. The Framingham Study. Circulation 61:1179–1182, 1980.

Hall, WD, and Wollam, GH: Systolic hypertension. Curr Probl Cardiol 7(6):7–40, 1982.

National Center for Health Statistics: Blood Pressure of Adults by Age and Sex, United States, 1960–1962. Vital and Health Statistics Series II, No. 4. U.S. Government Printing Office, Washington, DC, 1964, pp 1–2.

Hypertension in the Elderly

Richey, DP, and Bender, AD: Pharmacokinetic consequences of aging. Ann Rev Pharmacol Toxicol 17:49–65, 1977.

Vestal, RE, Wood, AJJ, and Shand, DG: Reduced beta-adrenoreceptor sensitivity in the elderly. Clin Pharmacol Ther 26:181–186, 1979.

MacLennan, WJ: Drug interactions. Gerontol Clin 16:18–24, 1974.

Blaschke, TF, Cohen, SN, Tatro, DS, and Rubin, PC: Drug-drug interactions and aging. In Jarvik, LF, Greenblatt, DJ, and Harman, D (eds.): Clinical Pharmacology and the Aged Patient. Raven Press, New York, 1981, pp. 11–26.

Greenblatt, DJ, and Shader, RI: Pharmacokinetics in old age: principles and problems of assessment. In Jarvik, LF, Greenblatt, DJ, and Harman, D (eds.): Clinical Pharmacology and the Aged Patient. Raven Press, New York, 1981, pp. 27–46.

Gifford, RW, Jr: Management of systolic hypertension in the elderly. Cardiovasc Clin 12:69–77, 1981.

Vestal, RE: Drug use in the elderly: A review of problems and special considerations. Drugs 16:358–382, 1978.

O'Malley, K, and O'Brien, E: Management of hypertension in the elderly. N Engl J Med 302:1397–1401, 1980.

Editorial: Hypertension in the over-60's. Lancet I:1396, 1980.

Messerli, FH, Glade, LB, Dreslinski, GR, Dunn, FG, Reisin, E, Macphee, AA, and Frohlich, ED: Hypertension in the elderly: haemodynamic, fluid volume and endocrine findings. Clin Sci Molec Med 61:393S–394S, 1981.

Kotchen, JM, McKean, HE, and Kotchen, TA: Blood pressure trends with aging. Hypertension (Suppl III)4:128–134, 1982.

Reidenberg, MM: Drugs in the elderly. Med Clin North Am 66:1073–1078, 1982.

------ 12 ------

MANAGEMENT OF COMPLICATED HYPERTENSION

The term *complicated hypertension* refers to the status of patients in whom high blood pressure has led to such complications as congestive heart failure or renal insufficiency, or in whom antihypertensive therapy makes the management of important coexisting disease, such as diabetes mellitus, more problematic, or who develop refractory hypertension (Table 12–1). In either case, the medical management of the hypertensive state is frequently difficult, and the patient may be at high risk for increased morbidity and mortality. Although space does not permit a thorough discussion of each of these entities, we will try to highlight some important points concerning the management of these patients.

MANAGEMENT OF THE PATIENT WITH COMPLICATIONS OF HYPERTENSION

The Patient with Congestive Heart Failure

Often the most rewarding hypertensive patient to treat is one with coexistent congestive heart failure. Successful blood pressure reduction with the appropriate medications usually results in marked improvement in cardiovascular performance. The unusual exception is the patient with irreversible cardiac damage (Table 12–2).

The Patient with Renal Insufficiency

The occurrence of hypertension in the setting of renal insufficiency sometimes constitutes an important therapeutic problem. The basis for the poor therapeutic results in managing such patients often resides in a lack of appreciation of the adverse effect of hypertension on renal function. A failure to correct moderate to severe hypertension usually leads to inexorable worsening of the renal failure and often to end-stage renal disease requiring dialysis. Even though the successful lowering of blood pressure is often associated with an initial transient decrement in renal function, the clinician must not back off at this point and accept hypertension as inevitable. Even if he must resort to temporary dialytic therapy in managing such patients, the hypertension war-

135

TABLE 12–1. COMMON STATES OF COMPLICATED HYPERTENSION

A. Those related to complications of hypertension or worsened by hypertension.
   1. Congestive heart failure
   2. Renal insufficiency
   3. Advanced peripheral vascular disease
   4. Cerebrovascular insufficiency
   5. Ischemic heart disease
B. Those related to the presence of an important coexisting disease
   1. Diabetes mellitus
   2. Chronic obstructive pulmonary disease
   3. Severe gout
C. Refractory hypertension

rants therapy because it still prevents the progression of cardiovascular disease and possibly prevents strokes. Additionally, several studies have indicated that the initial reduction in renal function is followed by improvement in glomerular filtration rate with a moderation of renal insufficiency (Table 12–3). Vasodilators such as hydralazine or minoxidil do not directly reduce renal blood flow. Recently, the question has been raised as to whether beta-blockers exert a *clinically important* adverse effect on renal function (see Chapter 6). There are insufficient data to answer this question, and these drugs certainly are not contraindicated in the patient with renal failure.

The Patient with Severe Ischemic Heart Disease

Again, good blood pressure control is imperative because it results in a decrease in the work of the heart. In selecting the agents for lowering blood pressure in such patients, it is important that the clinican avoid agents that might, by causing undue tachycardia, increase the oxygen requirement of the heart. As is also the case in patients with cerebral vascular insufficiency or severe peripheral vascular disease, one should avoid overly rapid or excessive decreases in blood pressure or postural hypertension (Table 12–4).

The Patient with Refractory Hypertension

In approaching such a patient, it is incumbent upon the clinician to ensure that the patient does not have a component of "office" hypertension, medication noncompliance, or pseudohypertension. Similarly, one should check for the use of pressor agents such as nasal sprays or for the presence of a secondary cause of hypertension, particularly renovascular hypertension.

When the above possibilities have been considered and excluded, the clinician should consider the possibility of so-called pseudotolerance, which is defined as a reversible loss of blood pressure control related to fluid retention.

TABLE 12–2. PHARMACOLOGIC MANAGEMENT OF HYPERTENSION IN PATIENTS WITH CONGESTIVE HEART FAILURE

1. Excellent blood pressure control is essential
2. Digitalis preparations usually indicated in acute phase
3. Diuretic almost always indicated
4. Avoidance of symptomatic hypokalemia is important
5. Beta-adrenergic inhibitors should be avoided; if required, they should be used in conjunction with digitalis and diuretics
6. Preferred sympatholytic agents are clonidine, prazosin, and methyldopa
7. Afterload reduction with hydralazine, minoxidil, or captopril may provide specific therapy of congestive heart failure

TABLE 12–3. PHARMACOLOGIC MANAGEMENT OF MODERATE TO SEVERE HYPERTENSION IN PATIENTS WITH RENAL INSUFFICIENCY

1. Blood pressure must be controlled, whatever the etiology of the hypertension
2. If hypertension is not controlled, severe renal failure is inevitable
3. Deterioration of renal function following blood pressure control is usually temporary
4. If serum creatinine concentration exceeds about 2 mg/dl (creatinine clearance less than approximately 40 ml/min), a loop-acting diuretic such as furosemide is often needed
5. Vasodilators such as hydralazine or minoxidil do not directly reduce renal blood flow
6. Whether beta-adrenergic inhibitors have a clinically important adverse effect on renal function is not clear

Figure 12–1 depicts in schematic fashion the postulated mechanisms underlying the phenomenon of pseudotolerance, whereby the blood pressure–lowering efficacy of vasodilating and adrenergic-inhibiting drugs may be blunted. As can be seen, the pivotal step is expansion of blood volume. As a consequence of the initial reduction of arterial pressure following the administration of either of these drugs, renal perfusion pressure is reduced, with a resultant retention of salt and water by the kidneys. Simultaneously, a decrease in hydrostatic pressure in the peripheral capillaries favors the translocation of fluid from the extravascular into the intravascular compartment. As a result of these two events, blood volume is expanded, and the blood pressure returns toward pretreatment levels.

Inadequate dosage of diuretics, nonadherence to dietary sodium restrictions, or both may contribute to pseudotolerance. A 24-hour collection of urine often enables the physician to assess sodium intake, since, in a steady state, despite the administration of diuretics, the rate of sodium excretion approximates sodium intake. Truly refractory patients tend to be seen more commonly in large city clinics. Typically, this is the type of patient whose therapy often requires a potent Step-4 agent, such as minoxidil or captopril (Table 12–5).

MANAGEMENT OF THE PATIENT WITH COEXISTENT DISEASE

The Patient with Diabetes Mellitus

Since hypertension and diabetes are so prevalent, it is not at all surprising that these conditions often coexist. Unfortunately for the patient, the hypertension often accentuates the tendency for accelerated atherosclerosis that is already present in the diabetic patient.

TABLE 12–4. PHARMACOLOGIC MANAGEMENT OF HYPERTENSIVE PATIENTS WITH SEVERE ISCHEMIC HEART DISEASE

1. Good blood pressure control important (decreases work of heart)
2. Avoid agents that might increase work of the heart, i.e., hydralazine or minoxidil (unless tachycardia obviated by concomitant use of sympatholytic agent)
3. Beta-adrenergic inhibitor is excellent Step-2 agent
   a. In rare instance of coronary vasospastic disease, cardioselective agent is preferable
   b. Avoid if congestive heart failure is present
4. Avoid overly rapid decrease in blood pressure, hypotension, or postural hypotension

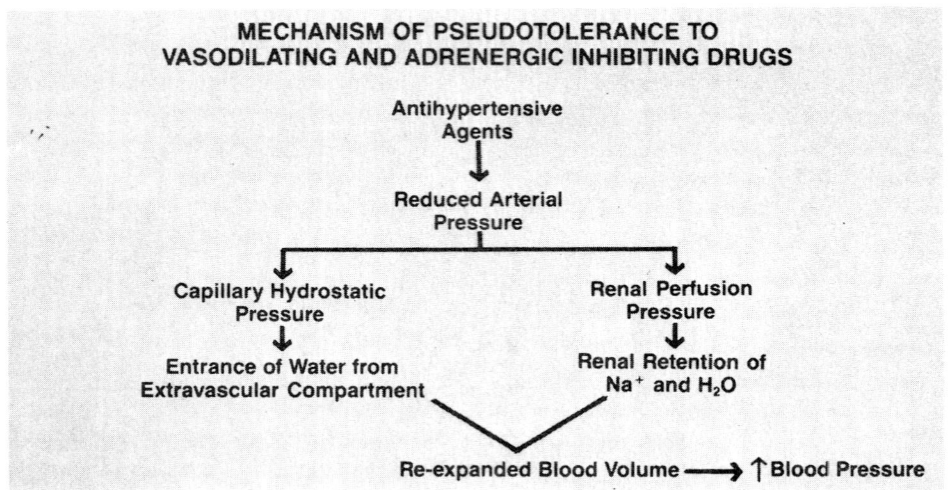

FIGURE 12–1. Schematic depiction of postulated mechanisms underlying the phenomenon of pseudotolerance, whereby the blood pressure–lowering efficacy of vasodilating and adrenergic–inhibiting drugs may be blunted. As can be seen, the pivotal step is expansion of blood volume. As a consequence of the initial reduction of arterial pressure following the administration of either of these drugs, renal perfusion pressure is reduced, with a resultant retention of salt and water by the kidneys. Simultaneously, a decrease in hydrostatic pressure in the peripheral capillaries favors the translocation of fluid from the extravascular into the intravascular compartment. As a result of these two events, blood volume is expanded, and the blood pressure returns toward pretreatment levels. (Reproduced with permission from "Management of Side Effects," from *Dialogues in Hypertension*. Vol. 4, No. 4, July 1982, p. 6. James C. Hunt, M.D., Executive Editor. Copyright 1982 by Health Learning Systems, Inc., Bloomfield, N.J.)

Although the need for therapeutic intervention is quite clear in diabetic patients, modifications of the antihypertensive regimen may be necessitated by the underlying diabetic state (Table 12–6). Thus, thiazide-type diuretics may worsen diabetic control. Conversely, potassium-sparing diuretics pose a distinct risk of hyperkalemia in the diabetic patient. As noted elsewhere (Chapter 6), this relates to hypoaldosteronism, insulinopenia, catecholamine abnormalities, and other factors.

Beta-adrenergic inhibitors may cause a masking of many of the symptoms of hypoglycemia, including tachycardia. Likewise, the duration of hypoglycemia may be prolonged and, when it occurs, paradoxical hypertension together with

TABLE 12–5. MANAGEMENT OF SEVERE HYPERTENSION REFRACTORY TO ROUTINE STEP-CARE

1. Does patient have a component of pseudohypertension or of "office" hypertension?
2. Try to exclude noncompliance; if pseudotolerance is suspected, a 24-hour collection of urine for sodium measurement can determine salt intake.
3. Does patient have an unsuspected secondary cause of hypertension, such as renovascular hypertension or pheochromocytoma?
4. Does patient have renal insufficiency or require a higher dose or a more potent diuretic for another reason?
5. Is patient offsetting antihypertensive effects of drugs with vasopressors such as nasal sprays or cold remedies, òr inhibitory drugs such as tricyclic antidepressants?
6. Have dosage of Step-2 and Step-3 agents been pushed to their maxima?
7. Patient may need to be started on a Step-4 agent, i.e., minoxidil or captopril. If hypertension is severe, hospitalization to initiate therapy with these drugs is often advisable.
8. If minoxidil and captopril fail, consider other agents, including nifedipine, guanethidine, phenoxybenzamine, and even repeated injections of diazoxide.

TABLE 12–6. PHARMACOLOGIC MANAGEMENT OF HYPERTENSION IN PATIENTS WITH DIABETES MELLITUS

A. Good blood pressure control is very important to lessen risk of complications related to accelerated atherosclerosis
B. Diuretics
  1. May exacerbate hyperglycemia
    a. By interfering with insulin release
    b. By producing potassium depletion
  2. Avoid use of potassium-sparing diuretics: spironolactone, triamterene, and amiloride
    a. Increased risk of hyperkalemia
C. Beta-adrenergic inhibitors
  1. Try to avoid, especially in insulin-requiring or hypoglycemia-prone patient
  2. Preferable to use cardioselective agent at lowest effective dose
  3. May mask some of signs of hypoglycemia: palpitations, tachycardia, and anxiety (but not sweating)
  4. Rarely, may prolong duration of hypoglycemia
  5. Rarely, may, in the presence of hypoglycemia, induce paradoxical hypertension, marked bradycardia, and intense peripheral vasoconstriction with cyanosis
  6. Rarely, may cause marked deterioration of diabetic control and even nonketotic hyperosmolar coma

peripheral vasoconstriction and bradycardia may result from relatively unopposed alpha-adrenergic receptor stimulation subsequent to epinephrine release. Finally, beta-blockers may result in a worsening of the diabetic state, with increasing hyperglycemia and, very rarely, hyperglycemic nonketotic coma.

The Patient with Chronic Obstructive Pulmonary Disease

The patient with chronic obstructive pulmonary disease is subject to both left- and right-sided congestive heart failure; control of hypertension may be extremely important. The clinician should avoid agents that may increase the work of the heart. As is the case with the diabetic patient, the use of beta-blockers can be fraught with potential complications, in this instance increased bronchospasm. Even though cardioselective agents, such as metoprolol or atenolol (or possibly ISA-positive agents), are less likely to produce this effect, selectivity is *relative* and diminishes considerably at the dosage levels frequently needed to control the blood pressure.

REFERENCES

Woods, JW, and Blythe, WB: Management of malignant hypertension complicated by renal insufficiency. N Engl J Med 277:57–61, 1967.
Woods, JW, Blythe, WB, and Huffines, WD: Management of malignant hypertension complicated by renal insufficiency. A follow-up study. N Engl J Med 291:10–14, 1974.
Kincaid-Smith, P: Malignant hypertension: mechanisms and management. Pharmacol Ther 9:245–269, 1980.
Tarazi, RC: Management of the patient with resistant hypertension. Hosp Prac, pp. 49–57, Jan. 1981.

ANTIHYPERTENSIVE AGENTS IN HYPERTENSIVE CRISIS

The preceding chapter has dealt with the pharmacologic approach to patients with mild to severe hypertension, entailing the use of *oral* antihypertensive medications. Fortunately, most patients seen by the practitioner will fall into this category. What about the patient, however, who has a hypertensive crisis, which demands that the blood pressure be lowered acutely? In such a setting, the approach to therapy must be quite different. Whereas with oral, outpatient therapy the emphasis is on gradual reduction of the blood pressure, in certain types of hypertensive crisis (see Chapter 2) the blood pressure must be reduced very quickly, although not precipitously.

Although the physician caring for the patient in hypertensive crisis has an armamentarium of several drugs for the management of this disorder, in recent years most intensive care physicians have relied largely on sodium nitroprusside and, to a lesser extent, on diazoxide. It should be emphasized that it is not enough merely to control the blood pressure acutely with these potent agents. Rather, it is mandatory that maintenance therapy with oral medications be initiated simultaneously.

Table 13–1 provides the reader with a listing of the agents that are currently in use for parenteral therapy of hypertensive emergencies. Medications, such as reserpine, that have fallen into disuse are not cited. The table also contains practical information regarding usual dose, route of administration, onset of action, times of maximal effect, duration of action, and major side effects. These topics, therefore, will not be detailed in the following discussion, whose purpose is to provide an overview and to stress the paramount principles of management.

Nitroprusside

In many ways nitroprusside is nearly an ideal agent for this condition. It acts almost immediately, and the offset of its antihypertensive effect is equally prompt. Used in sufficient dosage, it is practically always effective, and the blood pressure response can be titrated from minute to minute. The disadvan-

TABLE 13–1. DRUGS FOR PARENTERAL USE IN HYPERTENSIVE EMERGENCIES

Drug	Usual Dose	Route of Administration	Onset of Action	Maximal Effect	Duration of Action	Major Side Effects
IMMEDIATE-ONSET						
Diazoxide	5 mg/kg	Intravenous bolus*	1–2 min	2–3 min	3–12 hr	Tachycardia, angina, sodium retention, hyperglycemia
Sodium nitroprusside	0.5–3 μg/kg/min	Intravenous infusion	0.5–1 min	1–2 min	1–5 min	Nausea, muscular irritability, thiocyanate (and rarely cyanide) accumulation, methemoglobinemia
Trimethaphan camsylate	1–10 mg/min	Intravenous infusion	1–2 min	2–5 min	1–6 min	Ileus, urinary retention, cycloplegia
Phentolamine	5 mg	Intravenous bolus	Immediate	2 min	15–30 min	Tachycardia, hypotension, cardiac arrhythmias, flushing, nausea, vomiting, diarrhea
DELAYED-ONSET						
Hydralazine	10–20 mg	Intravenous or intramuscular	10–20 min	20–40 min	3–8 hr	Tachycardia, angina, headache
Methyldopa	250–500 mg	Intravenous	2–3 hr	3–5 hr	6–12 hr	Somnolence, parkinsonism

*Administration by repeated small bolus (50 or 100 mg) or drip infusion (5 mg/kg over a 20 to 30 min period) is also efficacious and minimizes hypotension.

tages of nitroprusside relate to the need for constant monitoring for the vital signs by the intensive care unit (ICU) nurse and the potential for thiocyanate and cyanide toxicity with prolonged high-dose usage, especially if the patient has renal or hepatic insufficiency.

Diazoxide

Diazoxide is also a very useful agent and, although not as consistently effective as nitroprusside, probably merits greater use. Relative to nitroprusside, its advantages are a prolonged duration of action, so that its administration may be intermittent, and a much smaller need (except immediately following administration) for constant blood pressure monitoring. Recently it has been recognized that diazoxide may be used efficaciously either by "slow" infusion (300 mg over 15 to 20 min) or by repeated "minibolus" (100 mg, given every five minutes as indicated). Use of the minibolus approach appears to reduce the risk of undesirable hypotension, which is more likely to occur in elderly patients and in those patients receiving other antihypertensive agents.

Disadvantages of diazoxide, relative to nitroprusside, are the inability to regulate the blood pressure from minute to minute, the occasional frank hypotensive reactions subsequent to its administration, and occasional resistance. In a patient with congestive heart failure (CHF) or low cardiac output syndrome, nitroprusside is clearly the preferred agent because of its beneficial actions on both cardiac preload and afterload without an undesirable increase in cardiac work.

Trimethaphan (Arfonad)

There is still a place, on occasion, for the use of the ganglionic blocking agent trimethaphan camsylate (Arfonad) in hypertensive crises. Although its mechanism of action is quite different, this medication produces prompt hemodynamic effects quite similar to those of nitroprusside and can be used in the rare patient who is "nitroprusside resistant" or in those patients in whom nitroprusside must be temporarily discontinued because of toxicity. Unfortunately, trimethaphan administration for more than one to two days is likely to be associated with some of the undesirable side effects of ganglionic blockade, including ileus, urinary retention, and cycloplegia.

Phentolamine

Phentolamine is an alpha-adrenoreceptor blocking agent that is believed to inhibit competitively both the postsynaptic and presynaptic alpha receptors (see Fig. 6–3). With regard to hypertension, its sole indication for parenteral use is for the acute reduction of marked increases in blood pressure in patients strongly suspected of having, or known to have, a pheochromocytoma. It is generally given as an intravenous bolus, and in a patient with pheochromocytoma the antihypertensive effect is immediate. The duration of action averages 15 to 30 minutes; repeat doses can be administered as needed. Phentolamine can also be given intramuscularly. Adverse reactions include hypotension, tachycardia, cardiac arrhythmias, weakness, flushing, nausea, vomiting, and diarrhea. In the event of a hypotensive reaction, the usual supportive measures, such as head-down position, are indicated. Of note, the specific countermeasure is the administration of norepinephrine; epinephrine in this setting may paradoxically produce a further fall in blood pressure.

Recently, there have been a number of reports and comments in the literature regarding the potential hazards of using potent parenteral antihypertensive agents in patients with severe hypertension. Apparently, precipitous and large (decrements in mean arterial blood pressure of 30 per cent or more) decreases in blood pressure carry the small but real risk of producing ischemic events, including blindness, cerebral infarction, and coronary insufficiency. Because of these sometimes disastrous, albeit quite uncommon, complications some investigators have narrowed their indications for the use of parenteral medications to those few situations (acute pulmonary edema, hypertensive encephalopathy, dissecting aneurysm, and unstable angina) wherein the immediate risk to life or to a vital end-organ justifies the potential hazards of therapy.

Oral Maintenance Therapy

We have noted that a difficult area for physicians is the approach to switching a patient from parenteral to oral medications following a hypertensive crisis. We offer the following suggestions.

1. Begin oral medications as soon as possible to avoid prolongation of the patient's stay in the intensive care unit and the need for parenteral medications.
2. Most, but not all, patients will require the use of multiple potent agents at high dosage. More often than the reverse, too-small doses are selected initially. Recently we have favored the use of a combination of at least two of the following types of agents:
   a. Diuretic—furosemide if the patient has renal insufficiency or is to receive minoxidil.
   b. Sympatholytic agent—clonidine or, if the patient has no CHF, bronchospasm, or other contraindications, beta-blocker.
   c. Vasodilator—hydralazine may be tried initially, and, if this is insufficient, minoxidil should be used. The role of captopril in this setting remains to be determined.

A brief summary of the course of a patient we treated recently is instructive.

The patient was a 21-year-old white woman with systemic lupus erythematosus and a history of severe complicated hypertension. Her regimen included digoxin, furosemide, propranolol, and minoxidil, but noncompliance was a serious problem. She was admitted to the medical intensive care unit following headaches and a generalized seizure, and was noted to have a blood pressure in the range of 220/150 mm Hg with papilledema. Serum creatinine levels were between 1.3 and 1.6 mg/dl. After two days' therapy with nitroprusside, 3 μg/kg/min; in addition to propranolol, 20 mg three times daily; plus furosemide, 20 mg twice daily; plus 30 mg of minoxidil over the preceding 24 hours, her diastolic blood pressure was in the range of 120 to 140 mm Hg. We were then consulted to aid in the management of her hypertension.

Because of probable hypervolemia and recent congestive heart failure, we recommended an increase in the dose of furosemide to 80 mg, twice daily; gradual discontinuation of propranolol; and addition of clonidine, with increasing dosage to a level of 0.5 mg twice daily, and minoxidil, 7.5 mg twice daily. The nitroprusside was tapered and stopped on the first day, and within two days the blood pressure averaged approximately 140/86 mm Hg without postural hypotension or deterioration of renal function.

Use of Medications other than Nitroprusside and Diazoxide for the Treatment of Severe Hypertension

When the blood pressure is very high (greater than 120 mm Hg diastolic) but the patient does not have a true hypertensive crisis (see Chapter 2), other agents can be used. There is still a place in this setting for intermittent parenteral administration of hydralazine given either intramuscularly or intravenously. Methyldopa can also be given by intermittent slow intravenous infusion.

Very recently a new form of therapy, clonidine loading, has also been reported. One regimen with which we have had successful results without hypotension is to give an initial dose of 0.2 mg followed by 0.1 mg hourly, up to a total dose of 0.8 mg or a reduction in diastolic pressure to less than 110 mm Hg. Arbitrarily, about 50 per cent of the total loading dose can then be given every 12 hours. Obviously, after the initial therapy, many such patients will also require a diuretic and a vasodilator such as hydralazine. This regimen should be used only in those patients for whom chronic clonidine administration is contemplated. Otherwise, withdrawal of medication might lead to a return of severe hypertension.

REFERENCES

Ram, CVS: Hypertensive encephalopathy. Recognition and management. Arch Intern Med 138:1851–1853, 1978.

Ram, CVS, and Kaplan, NM: Individual titration of diazoxide dosage in the treatment of severe hypertension. Am J Cardiol 43:627–630, 1979.

Ledingham, JGG, and Rajagopalan, B: Cerebral complications in the treatment of accelerated hypertension. Q J Med 58:25–41, 1979.

Anderson, RJ, Hart, GR, Crumpler, CP, Reed, WG, and Matthews, CA: Oral clonidine loading in hypertensive urgencies. JAMA 246:848–850, 1981.

Bertel, O, Conen, D, Radü, EW, Müller, J, Lang, C, and Dubach, UC: Nifedipine in hypertensive emergencies. Br Med J 286:19–21, 1983.

Beer, N, Gallegos, I, Cohen, A, Klein, N, Sonnenblick, E, and Frishman, W: Efficacy of sublingual nifedipine in the acute treatment of systemic hypertension. Chest 79:571–574, 1981.

Editorial: Dangerous antihypertensive treatment. Br Med 2:228–229, 1979.

MANAGEMENT OF SECONDARY HYPERTENSION

MEDICAL MANAGEMENT OF THE PATIENT WITH SECONDARY HYPERTENSION

As noted earlier, the optimal approach for the management of the patient with secondary (i.e., potentially "curable") hypertension is surgical correction of the abnormality, for example, removal of a pheochromocytoma, or revascularization of the renal arterial tree. Unfortunately, there are many instances in which such an optimal approach is not feasible because of concomitant disorders that preclude major surgery. The patient must then be treated medically and the question asked as to whether the pharmacologic approach differs in any way from that used in the patient with essential hypertension.

Although in general the medical management of patients with secondary forms of hypertension also uses the Step-Care approach, there are a sufficient number of differences to warrant specific comments concerning some of the entities, including renovascular hypertension (RVHT), primary aldosteronism, and pheochromocytoma.

Renovascular Hypertension

Many patients can be successfully operated upon, and some of those who are not deemed to be suitable surgical candidates may be treated by transluminal angioplasty. There is, however, a distinct subgroup in whom medical therapy is indicated. Patients with equivocal diagnostic results, or clinical and laboratory features known to reduce the chance of surgical relief (i.e., long-standing hypertension or extensive artherosclerosis elsewhere) may be initially treated medically. If such patients respond well, and if renal function does not deteriorate while they are under careful surveillance, medical therapy should be continued. Other patients that must be treated medically include those refusing surgery or considered at too high a risk because of coexistent serious disease.

Knowledge of the classification and natural history of renovascular disease is also important in the assessment of whether a patient is a surgical candidate. Each of the four different varieties of fibrous arterial disease has distinctive histologic and angiographic features and a different biologic history. In older patients with medial fibroplasia, medical management of hypertension can be safely advised, because progressive obstruction with loss of renal function does not usually develop in this setting. Conversely, in patients with renal artery stenosis due to intimal fibroplasia, perimedial fibroplasia, or true fibromuscular hyperplasia, progression and complicating dissections or thromboses are common. Furthermore, the hypertension in these patients is difficult to control, and renal revascularization should be performed as soon as possible, both to preserve renal function and to obviate the need for lifelong medical therapy.

The pharmacologic management of RVHT is basically the same as that of essential hypertension. Since RVHT is frequently characterized by severe (even malignant) hypertension, which is often refractory to therapy, the Step-Care approach, often eventually involving Step-4 agents, is well suited. To our knowledge, there are no convincing data that any one antihypertensive agent has prepotent efficacy in these patients. Nevertheless most investigators believe that beta-blockers constitute the initial drugs of choice because of their ability to decrease plasma renin activity (PRA). Finally, as mentioned above (see Chapter 6), initial observations indicate that inhibition of angiotensin-converting enzyme, even though often effective in decreasing the blood pressure, may be associated with a risk of reducing the glomerular filtration rate (GFR).

Primary Hyperaldosteronism

Although surgery should be carried out when the diagnosis is *adenoma*, treatment with spironolactone has a role in patients with adenomas who are unable or unwilling to have surgery, those patients who remain hypertensive after surgery, and those with equivocal findings. If the diagnosis is bilateral adrenal hyperplasia, only medical therapy is efficacious.

Once the decision to treat a patient medically has been made, the choice of the specific antihypertensive drug requires consideration. Medical therapy with spironolactone has a major role in the management of patients with primary aldosteronism. If thiazides alone are used, marked urinary potassium losses may result. Indeed, severe hypokalemia following thiazide administration often provides the initial clue to the diagnosis of primary aldosteronism.

Treatment with spironolactone usually is associated with persistent lowering of the blood pressure. After initiating treatment with doses of 300 to 400 mg a day, one may subsequently achieve a satisfactory response with much smaller doses. Combining small doses of spironolactone with a thiazide diuretic or amiloride sometimes provides even better control. Finally, in the patient (usually a man) who requires medical therapy but develops intolerable spironolactone-induced side effects, therapy can be instituted with a moderately restricted dietary sodium intake and a different potassium-sparing diuretic, such as amiloride or triamterene.

Pheochromocytoma

Both before and during surgery, or in patients in whom surgical cure is not feasible, drug therapy occupies an important role in the management of the patient with pheochromocytoma.

The two available alpha-adrenergic antagonists are phenoxybenzamine and phentolamine. These are useful not only for controlling blood pressure and allowing normalization of the contracted intravascular volume, but also for reducing sweating and improving glucose tolerance. Although both drugs may be administered orally, phentolamine, because of its rapid onset and relatively short duration of action, is usually reserved for intravenous use during a hypertensive crisis. Phenoxybenzamine is the preferred agent for long-term use and may be given twice daily in appropriately titrated dosages.

Currently, the only role for beta-adrenoceptor antagonists in the therapy of patients with pheochromocytoma relates to the treatment of tachyarrhythmias. Pheochromocytoma is the prototype of disorders characterized by a risk of beta-blocker–induced paradoxical increases in blood pressure, since the alpha-agonist property of epinephrine is relatively unopposed. Thus, beta-blockers should not be used until adequate alpha-blockade has been achieved. Similarly, the addition of a beta-blocker may require an increase in the dosage of alpha-blocker.

SURGICAL MANAGEMENT OF RENOVASCULAR HYPERTENSION

Once the patient with renovascular hypertension has been identified, consideration must be given as to whether he is a candidate for surgical intervention.

The attitude regarding renal vascularization for patients with atherosclerotic renovascular disease has been undergoing continuous reassessment in the last several years. Patients with atherosclerotic renovascular disease have long been considered a high-risk group for surgical therapy because of their age, frequently associated coronary, cerebrovascular, or peripheral vascular disease, and less satisfactory results when compared with patients with fibromuscular disease.

In this regard, the findings of the Cooperative Study of Renovascular Hypertension are of interest. The study assessed the blood pressure response to operative treatment of 502 patients. Fifty one per cent were cured, 15 per cent improved, and 34 per cent remained unchanged. At the time, renin determinations were not universally available to aid in patient selection, and postoperative arteriograms were not performed in all patients whose blood pressure failed to respond. Regardless, several points are clear. Patients with fibromuscular disease had a favorable blood pressure response (80 per cent) more commonly than patients with atheromatous disease (63 per cent). Moreover, patients with bilateral atheromatous disease had a less favorable response (56 per cent) and a high mortality (10 per cent). The overall mortality was 6 per cent, with a preponderance of deaths in patients with atheromatous disease (9.3 per cent), in contrast to those with fibromuscular disease (3.4 per cent). Analysis of data from the Cooperative Study indicated that the most important determinants of surgical mortality were coronary artery disease, bilateral renovascular disease, impaired renal function, and the complexity of the renal operative procedure. A recent study from the Cleveland Clinic has reported an extremely low operative mortality and morbidity, which were attributed to correction of existing coronary or cerebrovascular disease and reliance on methods of revascularization that obviate operation on a badly diseased aorta. Table 14–1 provides an overview of the important factors that militate for or against a favorable surgical outcome.

Recent reports from specialized centers using rigorous techniques for patient selection suggest that with appropriate selection criteria initial success rates may approach 100 per cent and mortalities range from 0 to 5 per cent. The relapse rate due to graft failure is approximately 20 per cent. More than 90 per cent of these failures occur within the first three months after surgery. Graft patency has been documented in some patients for as long as 20 years.

TABLE 14–1. FACTORS INFLUENCING THE OUTCOME OF SURGERY FOR RENOVASCULAR HYPERTENSION

Favorable Result	Unfavorable Result
Fibromuscular lesion	Atherosclerotic lesion
Localized unilateral segmental renal artery lesion	Extensive or bilateral renal and extrarenal lesions
Normal renal function	Decreased renal function
Age less than 50 years	Age greater than 60 years
Shorter duration of hypertension (<5 years)	Longer duration of hypertension (>5 years)
No associated disease	Associated important diseases, such as diabetes mellitus and coronary artery disease
Elevated renal vein renin ratio (>1.5)	Low renal vein renin ratio (<1.5)
Abnormal intravenous pyelogram	Normal intravenous pyelogram

Modified from Perloff and Schambelan: Clin Endocrinol Metab *10*:513–535, 1981.

Finally, there have been numerous advances regarding techniques for revascularization in patients with renovascular hypertension. A recent example is extracorporeal renal revascularization and autotransplantation (referred to as "bench" surgery). This method of treatment has been used in a small group of patients with hypertension caused by branched renal artery stenosis, all of whom would previously have been considered candidates for nephrectomy or nonoperative therapy. The advantages of performing extracorporeal revascularization include optimum exposure and illumination, a bloodless surgical field, greater protection from prolonged renal ischemia, and more facile employment of microvascular techniques and optical magnification. The removed kidney is flushed with Collins Intracellular Electrolyte Solution and is then submerged in ice slush saline to maintain hypothermia. In most cases, extracorporeal microvascular arterial repair is performed with a branched autogenous vascular graft, and the repaired kidney is then autotransplanted to the iliac fossa. Recently, Novick and associates at the Cleveland Clinic have claimed success with this approach in a small group of patients with extensive branched renal artery stenosis. Clearly, such an approach must be restricted to centers with surgeons who are highly skilled and experienced with this operation.

Nephrectomy vs. Revascularization

Although it is implicit that preservation of renal function is a major consideration in the surgical repair of RVHT, only recently have improved surgical techniques rendered it increasingly possible to repair stenosis without resorting to nephrectomy. In view of the distinct possibility that renovascular disease may develop in the contralateral kidney, preservation of kidney tissue is obviously the preferred approach.

After the decision has been made to treat RVHT operatively, the overriding consideration for the physician should be the availability of an experienced surgical team. Renal artery reconstructive surgery is a technically difficult procedure and, we believe, should be performed only by well-trained teams with considerable experience in many or all of the several surgical procedures now available (Table 14–2).

Percutaneous Transluminal Angioplasty

The development by Gruntzig of a double-lumen catheter with an expansile polyvinyl balloon has made percutaneous transluminal angioplasty a widely

TABLE 14–2. SURGICAL PROCEDURES USED FOR THE TREATMENT OF PATIENTS WITH RENOVASCULAR HYPERTENSION

1. Nephrectomy
    a. Total
    b. Partial
2. Segmental resection with end-to-end anastomosis
3. Aortorenal bypass graft
    a. Venous
    b. Arterial (e.g., hypogastric or splenic)
    c. Synthetic
4. Thromboendarterectomy
5. Intraoperative dilation
6. Renal reimplantation after microsurgery (auto transplant)
7. Percutaneous retrograde transluminal angioplasty

Modified from Perloff and Schambelan: Clin Endocrinol Metab 10:513–535, 1981.

used and respected technique. This procedure has now been used to correct lesions throughout the vascular system. Figure 14–1 depicts in a schematic fashion the technique of balloon dilation of an atherosclerotic lesion: The pressure of the inflated balloon fractures the plaque in the area of stenosis, stretching the vessel wall and expanding the lumen. In the past three years, several reports have appeared on the use of percutaneous transluminal angioplasty for treating both atherosclerotic and fibromuscular disease of the renal artery. This technique makes available potentially definitive treatment to many patients with RVHT who might not be appropriate candidates for major surgery. Patients who are inordinate surgical risks and those with pre-existing renal impairment, solitary kidneys, or posttransplant RVHT are most likely to benefit from this rather simple, convenient, relatively low-risk procedure.

The results to date suggest that percutaneous transluminal angioplasty may improve blood pressure control in patients with either atherosclerosis or fibromuscular disease, improve renal excretory function, and sometimes even restore renal function in patients with moderately advanced renal failure. The advantages over surgery include reduced cost, reduced morbidity, immediate

FIGURE 14–1. A schematic depiction of the technique of balloon dilation of an atherosclerotic lesion: The pressure of the inflated balloon fractures the plaque in the area of stenosis, stretching the vessel wall and expanding the lumen. (Reproduced with permission from "New Concepts in Treatment," from *Dialogues in Hypertension.* Vol. 4, No. 6, November 1982, p. 7. James C. Hunt, M.D., Executive Editor. Copyright 1982 by Health Learning Systems, Inc., Bloomfield, N.J.)

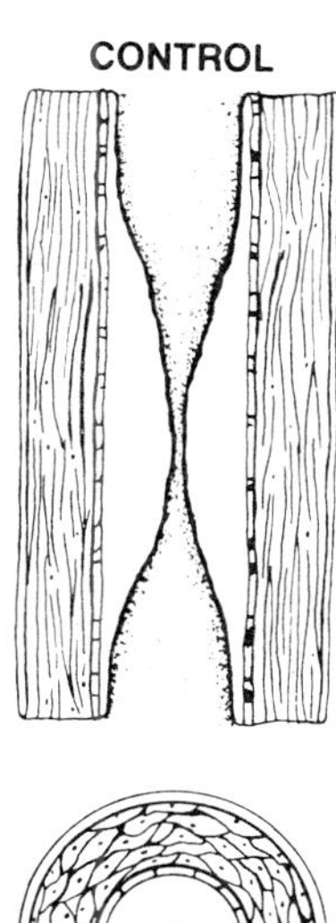

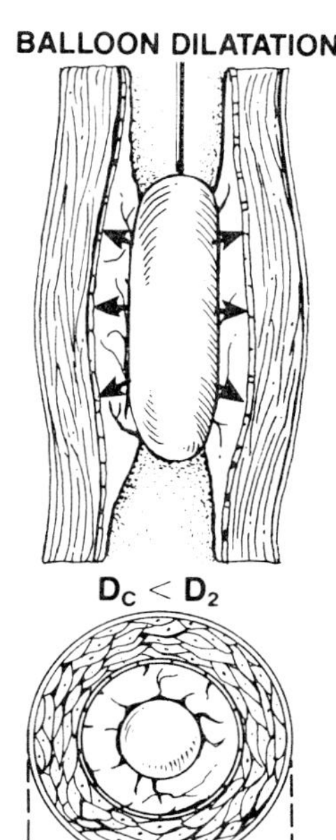

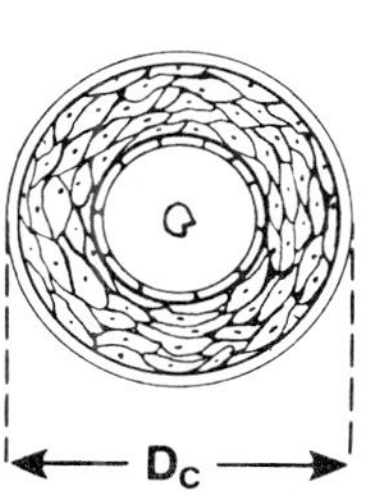

ambulation, and the fact that the procedure may be repeated easily. To date, several complications have been reported, including renal and peripheral embolization, femoral artery aneurysm, restenosis of a dilated artery, and contrast media–induced renal failure.

In a recent report, Grim et al. studied 26 patients with renovascular hypertension who were treated with percutaneous transluminal dilatation. Twenty-one were followed for more than one year; 18 underwent repeat angiography. Recurrence of stenosis was shown angiographically in one of six patients with fibromuscular disease and in 12 of 12 patients with atherosclerotic disease. The authors noted that the procedure was more likely to result in cure of hypertension (six of 10) in patients with fibromuscular disease than in patients with atherosclerotic disease (one of 16). In view of the unlikely but possible risk of serious damage to the renal vasculature by balloon dilation, it is recommended that a surgeon be on "stand-by" during the procedure.

Because of the relatively limited number of patients reported on and the rather short follow-up to this point, it is far too early to predict precisely what role this approach will come to play in the attack on renovascular hypertension. Although percutaneous transluminal angioplasty provides the advantages of simplicity, reduced cost, and probably reduced risk, the long-term utility of the procedure remains to be established. Ideally, a prospective randomized trial, the establishment of a registry, or both would serve to define more clearly the role of this therapeutic modality. Nevertheless, the advent of this moderately invasive approach and the promising early results indicate that transluminal angioplasty may loom as an important advance in the management of renovascular hypertension.

REFERENCES

Renal Artery Stenosis

Bookstein, JJ, Abrams, HL, Buenger, RE, Lecky, J, Franklin, SS, Reiss, MD, Bleifer, KH, Klatte, EC, Varady, PD, and Maxwell, MH: Radiologic aspects of renovascular hypertension. Part 2. The role of urography in unilateral renovascular disease. JAMA 220:1225–1230, 1972.

Novick, AC, and Straffon, RA: The current status of surgical therapy for renal artery disease. Am J Kid Dis 1:188–196, 1981.

Novick, AC, Straffon, RA, Stewart, BH, Gifford, RW, and Vidt, D: Diminished operative morbidity and mortality in renal revascularization. JAMA 246:749–753, 1981.

Case, DB, Atlas, SA, Marion, RM, and Laragh, JH: Long-term efficacy of captopril in renovascular and essential hypertension. Am J Cardiol 49:1440–1446, 1982.

Kaufman, JJ: Renovascular hypertension: the UCLA experience. J Urol 121:139–144, 1979.

Foster, JH, Dean, RH, Pinkerton, JA, and Rhamy, RK: Ten years' experience with surgical management of renovascular hypertension. Ann Surg 177:755–764, 1973.

Perloff, D, and Schambelan, M: Renovascular hypertension. Clin Endocrinol Metab 10:513–535, 1981.

Schrieber, MJ, and Novick, AC: Medical versus surgical management of renovascular hypertension. Cardiovasc Ther 12:93–106, 1982.

Novick, AC, and Stewart, BH: Surgical treatment of renovascular hypertension. Curr Probl Surg 16:1–16, Aug. 1979.

Novick, AC, Banowsky, LHW, Stewart, BH, and Straffon, RA: Renal revascularization in patients with atherosclerosis of the abdominal aorta or a previous operation on the abdominal aorta. Surg Gynecol Obstet 144:211–218, 1977.

Percutaneous Transluminal Angioplasty

Tegtmeyer, CJ, Dyer, R, Teates, CD, Ayers, CR, Carem, RM, Wellons, HA, Jr, and Stanton, LW: Percutaneous transluminal dilatation of the renal artery. Techniques and results. Radiology 135:589–599, 1980.

Novick, AC, and Straffon, RA: The current status of surgical therapy for renal artery disease. Am J Kid Dis 1:188–196, 1981.

Madias, NE, Ball, JT, and Millan, VG: Percutaneous transluminal renal angioplasty in the treatment of unilateral atherosclerotic renovascular hypertension. Am J Med 70:1078–1084, 1981.

McDonald, WJ: Renal artery stenosis causing hypertension: the current status of classical surgical therapy versus percutaneous transluminal dilatation. Am J Kid Dis 1:185, 1981.

Grim, CE: Percutaneous transluminal dilatation: the treatment of choice for renal artery stenosis causing hypertension. Am J Kid Dis 1:186–187, 1981.

Grim, CE, Luft, FC, Yune, HY, Klatte, EC, and Weinberger, MH: Percutaneous transluminal dilatation in the treatment of renal vascular hypertension. Ann Intern Med 95:439–442, 1981.

Primary Aldosteronism

Weinberger, MH, Grim, CE, Hollifield, JW, Kem, DC, Ganguly, A, Kramer, NJ, Yune, HY, Wellman, H, and Donohue, JP: Primary aldosteronism: diagnosis, localization and treatment. Ann Intern Med 90:386–395, 1979.

Ferriss, JB, Brown, JJ, Fraser, BR, Lever, AF, and Robertson, JIS: Primary hyperaldosteronism. Clin Endocrinol Metab 10:419–452, 1981.

Pheochromocytoma

Van Heerden, JA, Sheps, SG, Hamberger, B, Sheedy, PF, II, Poston, JG, and ReMine, WH: Pheochromocytoma: current status and changing trends. Surgery 91:367–373, 1982.

Falterman, CJ, and Kreisberg, R: Pheochromocytoma: clinical diagnosis and management. South Med J 75:321–328, 1982.

Atuk, NO: Pheochromocytoma: diagnosis, localization, and treatment. Hosp Prac 18:187–202, April 1983.

15

HYPERTENSION AND PREGNANCY

Hypertension associated with pregnancy constitutes a problem of major dimensions. It has been estimated that hypertension occurs in approximately one of 15 pregnancies. Hypertensive disorders of pregnancy account for approximately one fifth of maternal deaths and 25,000 stillbirths and neonatal deaths each year.

To approach this problem rationally a brief review of the profound changes in hemodynamics and hormones that occur during normal pregnancy is required.

As can be seen in Figure 15–1, blood pressure tends to fall during the early and middle portions of normal pregnancy, with a gradual rise toward, but not exceeding, nonpregnancy levels during the third trimester. The low blood pressures of normal pregnancy dictate that the criteria for what is "high" blood pressure be established at lower levels. The usual definition of hypertension during pregnancy is a sustained rise in blood pressure of 30/15 mm Hg, or any level greater than 140/90 mm Hg on two separate occasions. There is increasing evidence, however, that this cut-off point is too high. A task force of the National Institutes of Health examined the course of some 50,000 women and observed a marked increase in perinatal mortality when the blood pressure rose above 125/75 mm Hg before the 36th week. The perinatal mortality was even greater when pressures exceeded 135/85. We consider diastolic levels of 75 mm Hg in the second and 85 mm Hg in the third trimester as the upper limits of normal.

Classification of Hypertension in Pregnancy

After reading the literature dealing with high blood pressure and pregnancy, the clinician is often confused. In part, this is because investigators have often found it difficult to distinguish clinically between pre-eclampsia, essential or secondary hypertension, renal disease, and combinations thereof. Any cause of increased blood pressure may mimic pre-eclampsia. As an example of an uncommon but particularly confusing situation, the blood pressure of some women with undiagnosed essential hypertension may decrease early in gestation and be within the "normal range" when the patient is first seen near midpregnancy. This may lead to the erroneous designation of pre-eclampsia when the blood pressure subsequently increases near term.

It must be emphasized that the classification of hypertensive disorders is not merely an exercise of academic interest; rather, it is apparent that the rational management of the hypertension of pregnancy, as well as the prognosis for future pregnancies, varies with the specific diagnosis. The American College of Obstetricians and Gynecologists' Committee on Terminology has classified hypertensive disorders of pregnancy as

1. Pre-eclampsia/eclampsia
2. Chronic hypertension
3. Pre-eclampsia superimposed upon chronic hypertension
4. Late, transient, or "gestational" hypertension

Notice that the word *toxemia* does not appear in the classification. Since no hypertensive toxin has been discovered, the term is somewhat obfuscatory and no longer appropriate.

PRE-ECLAMPSIA

Pre-eclampsia usually develops after the 20th week of a first gestation, and most frequently near term, and is characterized by hypertension, edema, proteinuria, and at times disordered coagulation. When this disorder progresses to a convulsive phase it is termed *eclampsia*. Hypertension in the third trimester may be defined as a diastolic blood pressure of 85 mm Hg or greater sustained for 4 to 6 hours. Increments exceeding 30 and 15 mm Hg over earlier systolic and diastolic pressures, respectively, are considered abnormal, especially if the increases occurred rapidly.

Approximately 5 per cent of pregnant women develop pre-eclampsia. An increased risk is observed in women with multiple births, age greater than 35, hydatidiform mole, fetal hydrops, diabetes, Rh incompatibility, alpha-thalas-

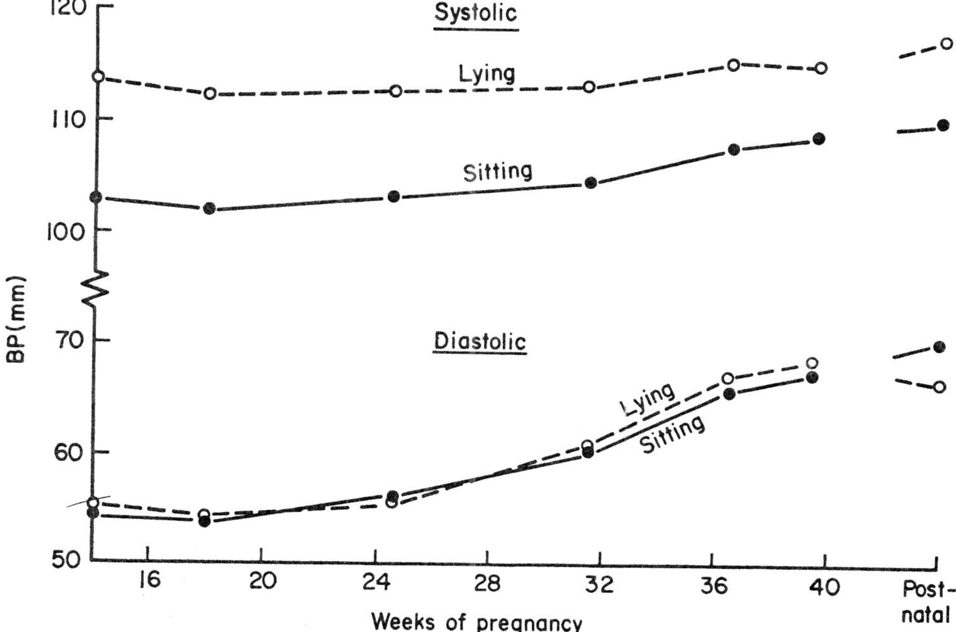

FIGURE 15–1. Alterations in blood pressure during normal pregnancy. As can be seen, blood pressure tends to fall during the early and middle portions of normal pregnancy, with a gradual rise toward, but not exceeding, nonpregnancy levels during the third trimester. (Reproduced with permission from MacGillivray, I, et al.: Clin Sci 37:395–407, 1969.)

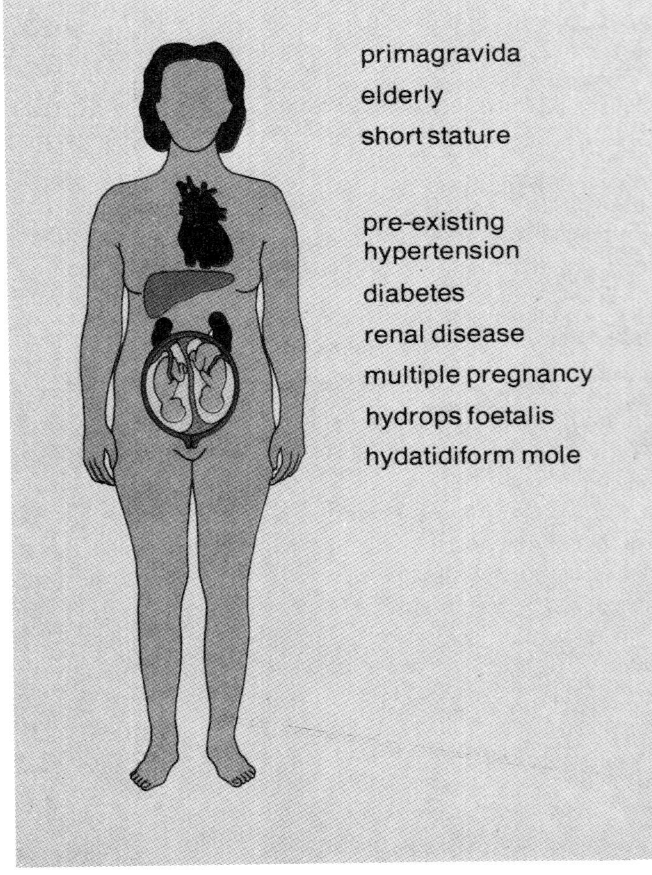

FIGURE 15–2. A schematic depiction of the principal factors that predispose women to pre-eclampsia. (Reproduced with permission from Hypertension Illustrated by WS Peart, PS Sever, JD Swales, and R Tarazi, courtesy of Gower Medical Publishing.)

semia, pre-existing renal disease with hypertension, teenage pregnancy, and a family history of pre-eclampsia. The principal factors that predispose women to pre-eclampsia are depicted schematically in Figure 15–2.

If pre-eclampsia is superimposed on chronic hypertension in a given pregnancy, it is likely to recur in a high percentage of subsequent pregnancies. Approximately one third of gravidas who develop pre-eclampsia during their first pregnancy become hypertensive during the subsequent pregnancy. Although controversial, it has been suggested that those women are from the population destined to develop hypertension in later life. On the other hand, women with a single episode of pre-eclampsia usually remain normotensive in later life. The incidence of pre-eclampsia is higher in black than in white women, but this may be related to the greater incidence of essential hypertension in blacks.

Proteinuria is characteristic of pre-eclampsia, and its degree generally correlates with the severity of the underlying renal lesion. The diagnosis of pre-eclampsia is suspect in the absence of proteinuria.

Because dependent edema may occur in as many as 50 per cent of normotensive pregnancies, it has limited diagnostic value. Nevertheless, the sudden appearance of edema of the *hands* and *face* during pregnancy should alert the clinician to the possible development of pre-eclampsia, since this is unusual during normal gestation.

The role of the renin-angiotensin system in pre-eclampsia is disputed. Angiotensin and aldosterone levels increase significantly during normal pregnancy, but the levels, if anything, are less increased with pre-eclampsia. An increase in pressor sensitivity to infused angiotensin II develops early in the course of the disease. Other factors postulated as important in the etiology of pre-eclampsia include decreased uteroplacental perfusion, abnormal coagulation, and immunologic injury.

Although the underlying etiology of pre-eclampsia is uncertain, a consistent feature of the disease is the development of glomerular endotheliosis with enlargement and obstruction of the glomerulus by increased cellularity.

Differential Diagnosis of Pre-eclampsia vs. Chronic Hypertension

Distinguishing eclampsia from chronic hypertension or hypertension of chronic renal disease may be difficult. Studies based on renal biopsy have shown that the clinical diagnosis is often incorrect. It has been reported that one fourth to almost one half of patients studied by renal biopsy turned out to have other hypertensive diseases, particularly chronic renal disease. In light of the frequency with which a misdiagnosis is made, attention should be focused on a number of features that favor the diagnosis of chronic hypertension with or without renal failure, rather than pre-eclampsia. These include the following:

1. Onset of hypertension before the 20th week of pregnancy
2. Absence of proteinuria and edema
3. Failure to develop hypertension during the first pregnancy, but its appearance in subsequent ones
4. Severe hypertension with end-organ damage, such as cardiac hypertrophy and retinal hemorrhages and exudates, suggesting chronicity
5. Age of 30 years or more
6. Failure of uric acid levels to increase

Renal Changes. To differentiate the above-mentioned entities, the clinician should be familiar with the changes attending a normal pregnancy. Normally, as a result of increased cardiac output and blood volume, glomerular filtration rate (GFR) and renal plasma flow are increased 25 to 50 per cent by the second trimester, and these changes persist to term. Similarly, the serum creatinine and blood urea nitrogen (BUN) concentrations usually fall during the last month of pregnancy.

Patients with pre-eclampsia sustain a reduction in GFR. Thus, their GFR, BUN, and creatinine may be in the normal range for a nonpregnant patient, but are inappropriate for a normal pregnancy. Most patients have negative urinary sediments, although a few will have microscopic hematuria and red cell casts. Significant hematuria is usually associated with underlying renal disease.

Other Changes. First, although often difficult to detect, retinal arterial spasm suggests pre-eclampsia, whereas arteriovenous nicking and hemorrhages and exudates are more characteristic of chronic hypertension. Second, the serum uric acid level may be useful: in normal pregnancy, the level is somewhat decreased because of enhanced urinary excretion. In essential hypertension, the level remains normal, and pre-eclampsia is characterized by hyperuricemia. In one study, uric acid concentration was observed to increase from 3.6 ± 0.7 to 6.4 ± 1.7 mg/100 ml. Unfortunately, sufficient overlap exists between the uric acid levels of these groups (and this is compounded by the hyperuricemic effect of diuretics) to limit the value of the determination. Finally, renal biopsy is the most definitive means of excluding chronic renal disease. Its risk must be weighed against its possible benefits, and if all the clinical and laboratory clues are considered, a correct diagnosis can usually be made without biopsy.

TREATMENT OF HYPERTENSIVE DISORDERS OF PREGNANCY

Prophylaxis

Since the optimal approach to pre-eclampsia is its prevention, much attention has been focused on measures that might lessen the risk of its occurrence. Unfortunately, nothing is known at present that safely prevents the occurrence of pre-eclampsia.

Many physicians advise their patients to gain less than 20 pounds during their pregnancy and to limit their salt intake. Some clinicians prescribe prophylactic thiazide diuretics to those who are most susceptible. Kraus et al., in a carefully performed study, found this to be of no benefit: The incidence of pre-eclampsia was identical (6.7 per cent) in 195 primigravidas who took 50 mg of hydrochlorothiazide daily during the last 16 weeks as in 210 who took a placebo.

In addition to the known complications of diuretic therapy (see pp. 71–77), diuretic-induced side effects, including hyponatremia and thrombocytopenia, have been reported in the infants as well.

Dietary Sodium Restriction

Although for many years obstetricians advocated the dietary restriction of sodium for both the prevention and therapy of pre-eclampsia, both the efficacy and the safety of salt restriction are of questionable value because

1. Sodium retention occurs in normal pregnancy
2. The occurrence of pre-eclampsia does not correlate with either the amount of weight gained or the presence of edema
3. No well-controlled studies are available bearing on the benefit (or lack thereof) of sodium restriction
4. Overenthusiastic dietary and diuretic therapy might lead to dangerous sodium depletion

At the present time a reasonable course would seem to be a compromise position of advocating neither a low nor a high salt intake. Certainly the prevention of pregnancy in young girls is justifiable, not only because they are most susceptible to developing pre-eclampsia but because they often eschew proper prenatal care.

Hospitalization vs. Ambulatory Treatment

As summarized in a recent review by Lindheimer and Katz, many clinicians believe that ambulatory treatment has no place in the management of pre-eclampsia, i.e., that suspicion of the disease is grounds for prompt hospitalization. Supporters of this viewpoint emphasize that the diagnosis of mild pre-eclampsia may be misleading, and seemingly stable patients can progress to eclamptic convulsions very rapidly. Thus, most authorities advocate hospitalization in order to diminish the frequency of convulsions and other consequences of diagnostic error and therapeutic inadequacy. Other workers have a less conservative outlook and, in a reliable, well-motivated patient, try outpatient therapy initially. The patient is instructed to remain most of the time in bed on her left side, which lowers blood pressure without producing hypotension. In addition, she is admonished to report immediately symptoms such as head-aches, right upper-quadrant pain, and visual disturbances. She should be seen twice weekly. Despite the above-mentioned caveats, moderate sodium restriction is usually advocated. Unreliable patients, those who have marked initial signs, and those not responding to treatment at home should be hospitalized to permit closer surveillance.

The severity of the syndrome and the nearness to term has an important bearing on the mode of therapy. In general, if the pregnancy is beyond gestation week 36 (corroborated by indices of fetal maturity), induction of labor is the therapy of choice, whereas attempts to temporize should be made if the gestation is at an earlier stage. Nevertheless, if blood pressures above 100 mm Hg diastolic persist after 24 to 48 hours of hospitalization, delivery is usually indicated regardless of the stage of gestation, since the mother is at risk and further attempts at temporization rarely save the fetus.

Antihypertensive Therapy

Fortunately, the majority of patients can be controlled by bed rest and sedation alone. If the above measures are unsuccessful, a percentage of patients will progress to severe hypertension, eclampsia, or both. For an extensive review of this topic, the reader is referred to the books of Gant and Worley and of Chesley, and to the recent chapter by Lindheimer and Katz. We will present only an overview on the pharmacologic management of this complication.

When antihypertensive agents are indicated, the available evidence, although limited, indicates that some agents are preferable to others. Ganglion-blocking agents, Rauwolfia derivatives, guanethidine, and converting-enzyme inhibitors should not be used, because of side effects either in the mother or fetus.

Hydralazine and methyldopa are the most frequently used agents in pregnancy. The latter is among the few subjected to controlled investigations, and it appears to decrease the incidence of midtrimester abortions. Despite a potential for embryotoxicity, clonidine is being used more frequently in Europe. Its use in late pregnancy appears safe and warrants further investigation.

Initial reports concerning beta-blocking agents were equivocal, and some authors stressed that these agents caused fetal bradycardia and hypoglycemia as well as intrapartum loss and small-for-date infants. Nevertheless, a number of more recent trials have been initiated. Their preliminary results are encouraging. One revealed that the outcome of pregnancy was better in the group receiving a beta-blocking agent than in the group receiving methyldopa.

Severe Hypertensive Crisis

When a hypertensive crisis occurs in a pregnant subject, only two antihypertensive agents are currently being used extensively: hydralazine (given parenterally) and, more recently, diazoxide. Unfortunately, administration of the latter may be associated with uterine atony; a very precipitous drop in blood pressure, which may jeopardize the fetus; and severe fetal hyperglycemia. For this reason, slow infusions of 30 mg, repeated as needed, may be preferable to the 300 mg dose often used in nonpregnant patients. Nitroprusside crosses the placenta and is potentially hazardous to the fetus. Fatal cyanide poisoning has been noted in experimental animals. Finally, although magnesium sulfate is the agent of choice for impending convulsions or frank eclampsia, it has little direct effect on the blood pressure per se.

The level of blood pressure to be achieved in this setting is somewhat controversial, as it is in other forms of hypertensive crisis. We favor aiming for a level of 90 to 100 mm Hg diastolic rather than attempting to achieve normal levels. In the last analysis, the mother's well-being often must take precedence over potential harm to the fetus.

REFERENCES

MacGillivray, I, Rose, GA, and Rowe, B: Blood pressure survey in pregnancy. Clin Sci 37:395–407, 1969.

Lindheimer, MD, and Katz, AL: Kidney Function and Disease in Pregnancy. Lea & Febiger, Philadelphia, 1977.

Chesley, LC: Hypertension in Pregnancy. Appleton-Century-Crofts, New York, 1978.

Page, EW, and Christianson, R: The impact of mean arterial blood pressure in middle trimester upon the outcome of pregnancy. Am J Obstet Gynecol 125:740–745, 1976.

Lindheimer, MD, and Katz, AI: Pathophysiology of preeclampsia. Ann Rev Med 32:273–289, 1981.

Lindheimer, MD, and Katz, AI: (guest eds.): The kidney in pregnancy. Kidney Int 18:147–278, 1980.

Fisher, KA, Luger, A, Spargo, BH, and Lindheimer, MD: Hypertension in pregnancy: clinical-pathological correlations and remote prognosis. Medicine 60:267–276, 1981.

Cockburn, J, Ounsted, M, Moar, VA, and Redman, CWG: Final report of study of hypertension during pregnancy: the effects of specific treatment on the growth and development of the children. Lancet I:647–649, 1982.

Chesley, LC: Hypertension in pregnancy. In Leventhal, JM (ed.): Current Problems in Obstetrics and Gynecology, vol. IV. Year Book Medical Publishers, Chicago, 1981, pp. 1–62.

Swartz, SL, Moore, TJ, and Schoenbaum, SC: Hypertension in pregnancy. In Hypertension. Contemporary Issues in Nephrology, vol. 8. Churchill Livingstone, New York, 1981, pp. 203–222.

Pipkin, FB: The renin-angiotensin system in pregnancy: why bother? Br J Obstet Gynaecol 89:591–593, 1982.

Lindheimer, MD, and Katz, AI: Hypertension and Pregnancy. In Genest, J, Koiw, E, and Kuchel, O (eds.): Hypertension, 2nd ed. McGraw-Hill, New York (in press).

Gant, NF, Jr., and Worley, RJ: Hypertension in pregnancy: concepts and management, Appleton-Century-Crofts, New York, 1980.

Redman, CWG: Treatment of hypertension in pregnancy. Kidney Int 18:267–278, 1980.

Kraus, GW, Marchese, JR, and Yen, SSC: Prophylactic use of hydrochlorothiazide in pregnancy. JAMA 198:1150–1152, 1966.

Illustrative Case Examples

CASE 1 DRUG INTERACTION: DIURETICS AND LITHIUM

A 58-year-old-man was given lithium carbonate for the management of psychiatric depression. Serum lithium levels were checked at appropriate intervals and were within the therapeutic range. Several months later the patient had his blood pressure measured as part of a physical fitness program available at his office, and it was found to be 160/100 mm Hg. Similar pressures were observed over the subsequent three-week period. Hydrochlorothiazide, 50 mg once a day, was begun, and the patient was advised to restrict his dietary intake of sodium. Approximately three weeks after initiation of diuretic therapy the patient's wife phoned his psychiatrist after she noted that the patient had developed signs and symptoms compatible with lithium intoxication, i.e., lethargy and confusion. He advised her to bring him to the emergency room, where laboratory analysis showed a serum lithium concentration of 7.0 mEq/L, a highly toxic level.

Discussion

This case report exemplifies a well-known, important drug interaction between diuretics and lithium.

Lithium is eliminated mainly by urinary excretion. The tubular handling of lithium is similar to that of several other substances in that contraction of the extracellular fluid volume is associated with a considerable increment in its tubular reabsorption. As a result, less lithium is excreted and the blood level may rise. It is not surprising, therefore, that the risk of acute lithium intoxication is considerably enhanced by the administration of diuretics. For this reason, the concomitant use of lithium and diuretics is relatively contraindicated unless carefully supervised by an experienced clinician.

CASE 2 DRUG INTERACTION: CLONIDINE AND TRICYCLIC ANTIDEPRESSANT

A patient's blood pressure was well controlled at 145/85 mm Hg with a long-acting diuretic, given once daily, and clonidine, 0.3 mg given twice daily. Following a death in the family, he developed a situational depression, which was treated by his neighbor, a psychiatrist, with amitriptyline. One week after beginning the use of this medication, he was seen in his physician's office, and a blood pressure of 175/100 mm Hg was observed. The amitriptyline was discontinued and supportive psychotherapy employed. The blood pressure gradually returned to the level of good control, and the emotional disorder proved to be transient.

Discussion

This case provides an example of a well-recognized drug interaction: the obviation of the blood pressure–lowering effect of a potent antihypertensive agent by an entirely unrelated medication. Tricyclic antidepressants have the potential of markedly blunting the antihypertensive efficacy of several drugs. This phenomenon was first recognized with guanethidine and later described for methyldopa and clonidine. The putative mechanism is interference with the uptake of the medication into its active site. Of interest, centrally acting sympatholytic agents such as clonidine may uncommonly exacerbate or provoke depression. In the present case, since the depressive episode appeared to be situational, the clinician chose to continue the clonidine, and no further problems ensued.

CASE 3 DRUG INTERACTION: FUROSEMIDE AND METOLAZONE

A 54-year-old man with long-standing, inadequately controlled, severe hypertension despite excellent compliance was seen in the clinic. His regimen consisted of furosemide, 160 mg; minoxidil, 50 mg; propranolol, 240 mg; and KC 120 mEq; all given twice daily. His blood pressure was 180/110 mm Hg. Because of the finding of 2+ pretibial edema, the decision was made to potentiate the natriuretic effect of furosemide with 2.5 mg per day of metolazone, in the hope of reversing a presumptive hypervolemic component of the resistant hypertension. The patient was given an appointment for the following week. On his return, he complained of generalized weakness, dizziness, and muscle cramps. Physical examination revealed a 10-pound weight loss, a standing blood pressure of 100/60 mm Hg, and diminished deep tendon reflexes. Whereas previously his serum electrolyte concentrations and BUN and creatinine levels had been within the normal range, they were now grossly abnormal: Na, 135 mEq/L; K, 2.1 mEq/L; HCO_3, 38 mEq/L; Cl, 82 mEq/L; BUN, 75 mg/dl; Cr, 2.5 mg/dl.

The patient was admitted to the hospital and initially treated with intravenous infusions of NaCl and KCl. After a four-pound weight gain, his blood pressure stabilized in the range of 150/90 mm Hg, and the BUN and Cr returned to 20 mg/dl and 1.4 mg/dl, respectively. He was discharged on a regimen identical to the above, except for the use of metolazone every five days instead of daily.

Discussion

This patient suffered from a not surprising complication of a therapeutic regimen—metolazone plus furosemide—that offers both unusual efficacy and great potential for adverse reactions. The physician probably was correct in his suspicion of a volume-related resistance to blood pressure control. This is not uncommon in a patient with severe hypertension who, in association with the use of minoxidil, develops sodium retention that is resistant to even very high doses of furosemide. Our approach to this problem would have differed somewhat. Because of the unpredictable risk of ECF volume contraction and fluid electrolyte abnormalities associated with the combined use of metolazone and furosemide, we believe that prudence dictates that such therapy be initiated in a hospitalized patient so that dosage and frequency can be altered appropriately on the basis of changes in blood pressure, weight, and laboratory data.

CASE 4 SIDE EFFECTS OF BETA-BLOCKERS AND ISA

A 53-year-old business executive was given propranolol 80 mg twice daily, along with chlorthalidone, 50 mg once daily, because of moderate hypertension. After several days he complained to his physician of a dramatically decreased ability to play tennis owing to rapid fatigability. He also noted intermittent dizziness at rest, occasional palpitations, and the sensation of cold extremities when in a cool environment. None of these symptoms had been present before he began antihypertensive therapy. Physical examination revealed a blood pressure of 140/85 mm Hg and a resting pulse of 42 beats per minute, which increased only to 54 beats per minute after rapid walking. Propranolol was discontinued, and pindolol 10 mg twice a day was begun immediately. The patient was seen again five days later. At that time the resting pulse was 68 beats per minute, which increased to 80 after rapid walking. He then began playing tennis again without noting early tiring. Likewise, the symptoms of cold hands and feet and occasional dizziness abated. Blood pressure control was unchanged.

Discussion

A not uncommon side effect of beta-blocker administration is reduced tolerance for exercise. This probably relates to obviation of the normal tachycardia-mediated increase in cardiac output attending vigorous exertion. In fact, athletic individuals should be cautioned about the possibility of easy fatigability after initiation of beta-blocker therapy. Should this occur, another type of antihypertensive agent that does not diminish cardiac output, such as prazosin, clonidine, or methyldopa, may be employed. In the present case, the patient displayed considerable bradycardia both at rest and after modest exercise. The former may have accounted in part for his symptom of dizziness. In addition, the patient noted cold extremities, one of the most common beta-blocker–related side effects, especially in a cold climate. This symptom probably is due to a decreased peripheral blood flow subsequent to the decreased cardiac output and perhaps to the increase in peripheral resistance associated with the administration of many beta-blockers.

The rationale for using pindolol (or oxprenolol) in such a patient is to take advantage of the intrinsic sympathomimetic activity (ISA) of these agents. Because these medications not only deny catecholamines access to beta receptors, but partially stimulate them, they appear to have a reduced tendency to induce certain undesirable changes, including resting bradycardia and reduction in skin temperature.

CASE 5 THIAZIDE-INDUCED HYPERCALCEMIA

A 47-year-old woman was given a thiazide diuretic for the treatment of mild hypertension. Two years previously, at the time of a cholecystectomy performed because of gallstones, the results of a biochemical profile were within the normal range. Approximately six months after beginning this therapy, she noted the onset of tiredness, anorexia, nausea, and constipation. These increased gradually in intensity, and she was hospitalized. The laboratory data were mostly normal except for a serum calcium of 14.7 mg/dl, a serum phosphorus of 1.7 mg/dl, and mild hypokalemia (serum potassium 2.9 mEq/L). Following discontinuation of the diuretic, the serum calcium declined somewhat (to 12.5 mg/dl), but not into the normal range, and the serum phosphorus and potassium levels increased to low normal values. Subsequent studies were consistent with the diagnosis of primary hyperparathyroidism. Following the removal of a single parathyroid adenoma the serum calcium normalized, and all the patient's symptoms disappeared.

Discussion

In comparison to hypokalemia, mild alkalosis, and hyperuricemia, hypercalcemia is a very rare adverse reaction to the administration of thiazide or thiazide-like diuretics. In patients without underlying abnormalities of calcium homeostasis, serum calcium levels may increase somewhat, but will only rarely exceed the upper limit of normal. The mechanism is believed to relate to a potentiation of the effect of parathyroid hormone (PTH) on bone and perhaps to the hypocalciuric influence of the drug. In patients with disordered calcium-phosphorus homeostasis, particularly primary hyperparathyroidism, the use of thiazides may unmask the underlying disorder by producing mild to moderate hypercalcemia. Similarly, already existing hypercalcemia may be markedly exacerbated. Of note, both hypokalemia and hypophosphatemia are well-recognized associations of both hyperparathyroidism and diuretic use (hypercalcemia is believed to impair the renal conservation of potassium).

CASE 6 BETA-BLOCKERS AND ASTHMA

A 23-year-old man was referred for management of recently discovered hypertension. Several blood pressure determinations were in the range of 170/95 mm Hg. There was a family history of hypertension and no clinical or laboratory evidence of a secondary cause. He complained of occasional episodes of tachycardia and palpitations. As a teenager he suffered from asthma, but no attacks had occurred within the last five years. In addition to an elevated blood pressure, physical examination revealed a regular pulse of 110 beats per minute and a few end-expiratory wheezes at the right lung base on forceful breathing. The patient was treated with a long-acting thiazide-like diuretic. After four weeks his blood pressure was 145/85 mm Hg.

Discussion

The patient described probably represents an example of hypertension associated with a hyperdynamic circulation in a young man. Sinus tachycardia is characteristic, and systolic hypertension often predominates. Hypertension in this setting generally responds nicely to the administration of a beta-blocker, which is considered by many to be the initial medication of choice. Nevertheless, it was considered (and appropriately so), that the clear-cut history of asthma was a strong contraindication to the use of this class of agents. Even though the risk of provoking bronchospasm in such a patient would be somewhat diminished by the selection of either a cardioselective or an ISA-positive agent, as opposed to propranolol, it would remain inordinate. Selectivity is relative and dose related. Too many alternate antihypertensive agents are available to warrant the use of beta-blockers for this purpose in patients with asthma, even if, as in the present case, no attacks have occurred for some time.

CASE 7 DISCONTINUATION SYNDROME

A 57-year-old man with a long history of uncomplicated hypertension was hospitalized because of severe headaches and blurred vision of one day's duration. His most recent antihypertensive regimen consisted of chlorthalidone, 50 mg once daily; propranolol, 80 mg twice daily; and clonidine, 0.8 mg twice daily. Two days before admission the patient misplaced his supply of clonidine without seeking another source, but continued to take the other medications. There was no prior history of hypertensive crisis. Physical examination revealed a blood pressure of 220/130 mm Hg, retinal arteriolar spasm, and early papilledema. Mental status was normal, and there was no evidence of congestive heart failure or focal neurologic deficits. The patient was treated with bed rest, and clonidine therapy was reinstituted, using an acute-loading regimen (see p. 144). After six hours the blood pressure was 160/90 mm Hg, and the headaches had abated. He was discharged on his old regimen with the admonition to avoid abrupt discontinuation of any of his medications.

Discussion

This case exemplifies a severe instance of the discontinuation syndrome. Since the patient had no prior history of severe hypertension, it probably represents a genuine case of overshoot hypertension, which fortunately is quite uncommon. As discussed in the text, the most important predisposing factors were probably the abrupt termination of the relatively high dose of the centrally acting sympatholytic agent clonidine and perhaps the concomitant use of the beta-blocker propranolol. It is believed that beta-blockers (particularly those of the noncardioselective type) enhance the risk of the discontinuation syndrome by leaving the typical postwithdrawal-increased alpha-adrenergic activity relative unopposed. Characteristically, reinstitution of clonidine therapy resulted in resolution of the syndrome. If the situation had been more urgent, nitroprusside or the alpha-blocking medication phentolamine would have been indicated.

CASE 8 MILD HYPERTENSION

A 45-year-old asymptomatic white business executive underwent a routine medical evaluation as part of a physical fitness program sponsored by his employer. He admitted to a 15 pack-year history of smoking. His blood pressure was noted to be 140/95 mm Hg, and this level was confirmed on several subsequent determinations. He was not overweight. Laboratory studies documented the absence of electrocardiographic evidence of left ventricular hypertrophy, hypercholesterolemia, and glucose intolerance. The patient was referred to an internist as a possible candidate for medical therapy.

Discussion

Data accumulated from the Framingham Study indicate that a man of this age with either a systolic blood pressure of 165 or a diastolic blood pressure of 95 mm Hg has only approximately a 1 per cent increased risk of incurring a myocardial infarction over a six-year period, if no other risk factors are present. Contrariwise, the coexistence of all of the above-mentioned factors increases the risk to about 25 per cent, and the increase in risk attributable to hypertension per se is 6.6 per cent. Of interest, the statistically predictable benefit from discontinuaton of smoking is similar to that achievable by reduction of the blood pressure to normal. The recommendation of the patient's physician was to cease smoking, avoid excessive salt ingestion, begin a program of moderate exercise, and return to the physician's office periodically for follow-up blood pressure measurement.

CASE 9 MILD HYPERTENSION: CARDIOPROTECTION BY BETA-BLOCKERS

A 50-year-old black man returned to his hometown three weeks after suffering a subendocardial myocardial infarction while on a fishing trip. Three years previously, he had been found to have mild hypertension (blood pressures in the range of 155/95 mm Hg). At the doctor's office, the blood pressure when taken several times was also in this range. The patient had no angina and was asymptomatic. He planned to return to his work as an office manager in another three weeks. Aside from coronary artery disease, there was no clinical evidence of end-organ dysfunction. Timolol, 10 mg twice a day, was prescribed. Two weeks later the blood pressure was 140/85 mm Hg, and there were no apparent side effects.

Discussion

The patient had recently experienced a myocardial infarction. This evidence of end-organ dysfunction justifies antihypertensive therapy in a patient with mild hypertension. Furthermore, the described scenario affords the physician the opportunity of taking advantage of one of the so-called additional salutary effects of certain antihypertensive agents, in this case a beta-blocker. As discussed in the text, although the controversy regarding diuretics versus beta-blockers still rages, when the patient in question has recently experienced a myocardial infarction it makes sense to use the latter and thereby incur the added benefit of a reduction of the risk of a sudden arrhythmic death or a second ischemic event. Beta-inhibitors other than timolol have also been shown to be cardioprotective. Although beta-blockers tend to be less effective in black patients, this obviously need not be a major consideration in an individual patient.

CASE 10 NONDIURETIC MONOTHERAPY

During a routine insurance examination, a 30-year-old college instructor was discovered to be hypertensive. Blood pressures taken on several occasions were in the range of 170/105 mm Hg. There was no clinical or laboratory evidence of curable hypertension. The patient was given guanabenz at a starting dose of 4 mg twice daily. Initially he noted drowsiness and dry mouth but stated that after one week these symptoms abated. Two weeks after initiation of therapy his blood pressure was 160/100 mm Hg. The dosage was increased to 8 mg twice daily. Two weeks later the blood pressure was 150/95 mm Hg, but the previously noted side effects had reappeared. When the dosage was further increased to 12 mg twice a day, the response was better, but normotension (140/85 mm Hg) was not achieved until a regimen of 16 mg twice a day was used, and this dose was associated with persistent intolerable sleepiness and dry mouth.

Discussion

This case exemplifies a number of problems and controversial areas regarding the pharmacologic management of hypertension. The physician caring for the patient decided to use nondiuretic monotherapy. As discussed in the text, this appears to be a valid approach, although, except for beta-blockers, the reported experience at present is quite limited. The potential advantages of monotherapy include simplicity and avoidance of some of the metabolic side effects of diuretics. Some of the potential disadvantages of monotherapy were observed in this patient. First, the titration process was not easy, and it required three dosage changes before control was achieved. Second, a relatively high dose of the agent was needed; this increased the chance of side effects and obviously increased the cost. Somewhat surprisingly, it is frequently not feasible to normalize blood pressure with one agent, even in patients with mild hypertension. Unfortunately, drowsiness and dry mouth are relatively common offensive side effects of centrally acting sympatholytic agents. Although these tend to diminish with continuing use of the medication, they are also dose related, and with high dosage a substantial percentage of patients will prove noncompliant because of adverse reactions.

In this particular patient, the simplest approach to the problem would be to reduce the dose of guanabenz and begin administering a long-acting diuretic.

CASE 11 IMPOTENCE WITH THIAZIDES, AND NONCOMPLIANCE

A 47-year-old white construction worker was noted to be hypertensive during routine examination. He was referred to his physician, who, following an appropriate evaluation, started the patient on hydrochlorothiazide in a dose of 50 mg twice daily. The patient's blood pressure was well controlled during the subsequent six months. He returned for re-evaluation at nine months, at which time he was noted to again be hypertensive, with a blood pressure of 168/97 mm Hg. In light of the loss of control, the physician astutely queried the patient regarding changes in life-style or dietary sodium intake and asked whether he was compliant. Following repeated questioning, the patient admitted that he had discontinued the medication because of impotence.

Discussion

Inhibitors of the sympathetic nervous system may cause impotence, and in some instances a causal relationship has been supported by rechallenge. In contrast, although decreased libido has been attributed to thiazide diuretics, the association between these agents and impotence has only recently been substantiated. The mechanism whereby thiazide-like drugs may cause impotence is unclear, but it might relate to a decline in peripheral vascular resistance.

This case emphasizes the importance of side effects as a determinant of compliance with an antihypertensive regimen. Whenever there is an apparent lack of response to drugs, it is mandatory that the clinician question the patient to ascertain if there is noncompliance because of important side effects.

CASE 12   DRUG INTERACTION: BETA-BLOCKERS AND SYMPATHOMIMETIC NOSE DROPS

The hypertension of a patient whose untreated blood pressure was 170/100 mm Hg was nicely controlled for several months (blood pressures in the range of 140/80 mm Hg) with hydrochlorothiazide, 50 mg, and propranolol, 80 mg, both given twice daily. When the hay fever season began, without telling his physician, the patient began to use phenylephrine nose drops three or four times a day to relieve nasal congestion. After approximately four days, he noted frequent headaches, sometimes of a throbbing nature. An office visit disclosed a blood pressure of 180/115 mm Hg. Discontinuation of the nose drops and a few days of rest resulted in a return of excellent blood pressure control.

Discussion

This case exemplifies an important interaction—a marked increment in blood pressure following the use of sympathomimetic agents (in this case the alpha-adrenergic agonist phenylephrine) in patients receiving a beta-blocker. Sympathomimetic nose drops or sprays obviously may produce hypertension in their own right, but the risk appears to be markedly enhanced by concomitant beta-blockade, since alpha receptor stimulation becomes relatively unopposed. Although the likelihood of this interaction is probably diminished by the use of cardioselective agents, which have a lesser tendency to inhibit the beta-2 receptor in arteriolar walls, the risk is not eliminated. Patients receiving beta-blockers or any other antihypertensive medications should not take any new drug, over-the-counter or otherwise, without notifying their physician.

CASE 13   CAPTOPRIL: TEST-DOSE METHOD OF INITIATING THERAPY

The hypertension of a 42-year-old diplomat was poorly controlled in spite of adequate compliance with large doses of clonidine, hydralazine, and furosemide. Blood pressures, lying and sitting, were consistently at the level of 180/115 mm Hg. In addition, the patient had left ventricular hypertrophy and strain by ECG, cardiomegaly on x-ray, and mild renal insufficiency. The patient was referred to a nephrologist for his opinion. It was decided to treat the patient's resistant hypertension aggressively, particularly in view of the good evidence of end-organ damage.

The advisability of a short hospitalization to facilitate the safe initiation of captopril therapy was discussed with the patient, but he refused on the grounds of important commitments. The patient agreed, however, to spend the better part of a morning in the office. While continuing his prior medications, he was given a 6.25-mg test dose of captopril. Two hours later his blood pressure had declined modestly to 170/104 mm Hg.

He was sent home with instructions to add captopril, 6.25 mg three times a day, to his pre-existing regimen and to report any adverse effects immediately. Three days later he was seen in the office. The blood pressure was 165/100 mm Hg. The dose of captopril was increased to 12.5 mg three times daily. A week later, the blood pressure—lying, standing, and following brisk walking—was 155/95 mm Hg.

Discussion

Unfortunately, the most efficacious medications often possess substantial potential risks. Such may be the case with captopril. Presently, although this may represent an overrestriction, the current recommendation of the FDA and the manufacturer is that the use of captopril be limited to patients with resistant hypertension.

Particularly in patients receiving other potent antihypertensive agents coterminously, captopril, like prazosin, has the potential for inducing a first-dose hypotensive reaction. Furthermore, as is the case with minoxidil and other medications, renal function may decline in association with marked and excessive decrements of blood pressure. Mainly because of the risk of hypotension and its attendant adversities in patients with severe hypertension, it is prudent, although not always necessary, to begin captopril during hospitalization. Furthermore, the potential risk for marked increases in blood pressure frequently renders it inadvisable, in the patient with severe hypertension, to withdraw other medications before starting captopril, even though this course of action is recommended by the manufacturer and is theoretically ideal.

The patient under discussion refused admission to the hospital. We concur with the compromise solution employed by his physician to use a small test dose of 6.25 mg followed by close monitoring. The 25-mg tablets are conveniently scored to facilitate division into either two or four pieces. In the case example, blood pressure control was much improved with the use of captopril, 12.5 mg three times a day. At that point, slow tapering of the dosage of the other agents (and possibly eventual discontinuation of some of them), one at a time, would be warranted. If necessary, the dose of captopril could then be increased. Of interest, preliminary reports suggest that, for some patients at least, a dosing regimen of only 25 mg three times a day may be as efficacious as much larger doses.

CASE 14   CHOICE OF A STEP-1 DRUG

A 34-year-old engineer was referred for management of recently discovered hypertension. Several blood pressure determinations were in the range of 148/102 mm Hg. There was no family history of hypertension and no clinical or laboratory evidence of a secondary cause. Because of recent advertisements in medical journals suggesting that the centrally acting sympatholytic agents may constitute appropriate Step-1 medications, his physician initiated treatment with clonidine in an initial dose of 0.1 mg twice daily. When this was later increased to 0.3 mg, the patient's wife phoned the physician to complain that her husband was somnolent to the point that he was unable to report to his job. Clonidine was gradually discontinued and therapy reinitiated with the beta-blocker nadolol, starting with a dose of 80 mg once a day. The dose was increased when the patient was reassessed two weeks later. At the time of re-examination, the blood pressure was adequately controlled, being in the range of 138/86 mm Hg. The patient was no longer somnolent, and he was able to once again function without impairment in his role as a supervisor.

Discussion

As noted in the chapter on pharmacologic therapy (Chapter 6), the consensus is that either a diuretic or a beta-blocker should be selected as the Step-1 drug. Recently, a minority opinion has emerged suggesting that clonidine and other agents may also be useful as monotherapy in the management of hypertension. Although it may be efficacious in some cases, the dose of clonidine necessary to control blood pressure is often sufficiently large that (as exemplified by the present case) severe side effects, prominently lethargy and somnolence, ensue.

Notice that once the decision for discontinuation was made, the physician took the precaution of *gradually tapering* this agent to reduce the risk of a withdrawal syndrome. He then selected a beta-blocker with properties tending to minimize central nervous system side effects. Nadolol is a water-soluble beta-adrenoceptor blocking agent that penetrates the CNS poorly. Consequently, CNS side effects appear to be less often encountered than with more lipophilic agents (see p. 83).

CASE 15   DIURETICS IN PATIENTS WITH RENAL INSUFFICIENCY

A 38-year-old man was referred for management of recently discovered hypertension. Several blood pressure determinations were in the range of 150/94 mm Hg. In addition to the elevated blood pressure, there was significant pitting edema of the lower extremities. Routine laboratory data disclosed a normal CBC but abnormal blood chemistries: The BUN was 47 mg/dl, and the serum creatinine 3.3 mg/dl. A creatinine clearance was not determined. Treatment was initiated with a long-acting thiazide-type diuretic, and the patient was instructed to return to the physician's office in two weeks for re-evaluation. At the time of re-examination, the patient was still hypertensive, with blood pressure noted again to be in the range of 145–150/94–98 mm Hg. In an attempt to ascertain whether the patient complied with instructions, he was questioned as to his adherence to the prescribed regimen. The patient insisted that he had been taking the prescribed medication twice daily as instructed.

A nephrologic consultation was obtained, and a 24-hour endogenous creatinine clearance was determined, disclosing a creatinine clearance of 26 ml/min. The thiazide diuretic was discontinued, and the loop diuretic furosemide was substituted at a dose of 20 mg twice daily. In addition, the patient was instructed to restrict his dietary sodium intake, with prohibition of all "added salt." A re-examination two weeks later disclosed disappearance of the edema and a marked amelioration of his hypertension, with a decrease in the blood pressure to 134/90 mm Hg.

Discussion

Although diuretic therapy constitutes a rational choice for a Step-1 drug, the efficacy of such therapy depends in part on underlying renal function. Both thiazide diuretics and the more potent loop diuretics are equally effective in lowering blood pressure in patients with relatively preserved renal function. In fact, the former are preferred because of a lower risk of inducing fluid and electrolyte abnormalities. Nevertheless, when renal function declines so that the GFR (as assessed by the creatinine clearance) falls below 25 to 35 ml/min, thiazide diuretics are relatively ineffective, and loop diuretics may be required. If an initial laboratory determination discloses modest azotemia, the clinician should entertain the possibility that the GFR is diminished and measure endogenous creatinine clearance. The subsequent choice of a diuretic should be predicated on such a determination. As exemplified in this case, when the thiazide diuretic was discontinued and a loop diuretic initiated, edema was mobilized, and the blood pressure was effectively lowered. The consultant's suggestion that sodium intake be restricted concomitantly may have contributed to the salutary results. It must be emphasized that even if the appropriate diuretic is selected, it may prove ineffective if dietary sodium intake is sufficiently excessive. Continued ingestion of excess dietary sodium may counteract the salutary effects of even potent diuretics, thereby resulting in a "drug failure."

CASE 16   PSEUDOHYPERTENSION

A 63-year-old woman was admitted to the hospital because of an extremely high blood pressure associated with two days of intermittent headache. She had a ten-year history of mild hypertension. Physical examination revealed the patient to be alert and in no distress. The blood pressure was 260/170 mm Hg in both arms and was unchanged by posture. The fundi showed arteriolar narrowing without hemorrhages, exudates, or papilledema. There were no signs of congestive heart failure, no abdominal bruits, and no evidence of neurologic deficits. The peripheral pulses were diminished, but a thickening of the vessels could not be appreciated.

Laboratory data included a normal BUN and serum creatinine. Neither the chest x-ray nor the ECG showed evidence of cardiomegaly or left ventricular hypertrophy. Because of the extraordinarily high blood pressure, the patient was placed in the MICU. When two intramuscular injections of hydralazine failed to alter the blood pressure, an infusion of nitroprusside was begun, with a similar apparent lack of efficacy despite the use of very high dosages. The blood pressure, both by cuff and Doppler instrumentation, remained in the range of 250/165 mm Hg. A nephrologic consultation was sought. The nephrologist emphasized strongly the need for determination of the intra-arterial pressure. When the MICU resident was unable to place an "A-line," a surgeon was called. With difficulty, he was able to thread a catheter into a markedly thickened radial artery. There was very little blood flow. The pressure within this vessel was 110/70 mm Hg; a simultaneously measured pressure by cuff was 240/150 mm Hg. An intra-arterial axillary artery pressure was obtained in order to confirm the accuracy of the radial artery determination. There was good agreement. Nitroprusside administration was discontinued immediately; the A-line pressure increased to 150/90 mm Hg. The headache disappeared on the second hospital day; its etiology remained uncertain.

Discussion

The case history of this patient (whom we encountered recently) is an excellent example of *pseudohypertension* (see Chapter 1). A suggestive clue to this diagnosis was the extraordinarily high blood pressure in the absence of evidence of end-organ damage on physical examination or laboratory investigation. Even if the severe hypertension were of relatively sudden onset (as from an intracranial hemorrhage) the patient would have had more symptoms and signs than a rather mild headache. Finally, complete resistance to nitroprusside is extremely unusual.

One of the important points to be emphasized is that therapy (especially the parenteral administration of as potent an agent as nitroprusside) for pseudohypertension is obviously inappropriate and potentially hazardous. We once saw a similar patient develop severe prerenal azotemia and obtundation from unrecognized nitroprusside-induced hypotension.

Unfortunately, there is no way to know in advance if a given patient has pseudohypertension. It probably is a common cause of apparent elevation of both systolic and diastolic blood pressure (or further elevation of a mildly increased blood pressure) in the elderly. Whereas some of these patients have palpably thickened, occasionally rock-hard arteries (particularly brachial), and soft-tissue x-rays of the extremities may show calcified, pipelike vessels, this may not be the case.

CASE 17 MISMANAGEMENT OF SEVERE HYPERTENSION

A 54-year-old man with probable renovascular hypertension was not considered an operative candidate and was being treated medically. He had been admitted to the hospital on two previous occasions because of hypertensive crisis. In spite of good compliance and the prolonged daily use of furosemide, 160 mg; clonidine, 1.2 mg; and minoxidil, 40 mg, his blood pressure was 180/100 mm Hg, and he was hospitalized for better control. He was asymptomatic. Physical examination revealed a blood pressure of 175/105 mm Hg, hard retinal exudates, and no evidence of congestive heart failure or fluid overload. Serum creatinine and electrolyte levels were within the normal range.

On admission, minoxidil was discontinued. Clonidine was withdrawn over the next 24 hours, and captopril, 25 mg twice a day, was begun. On the second hospital day, the blood pressure was 145/95 mm Hg, but thereafter, despite increments in the dosage of captopril to 450 mg per day and the initiation of therapy with propranolol, 240 mg per day, the pressure increased to the range of 200–220/135–150 mm Hg. He was transferred to the MICU, where nitroprusside (in addition to the above-mentioned oral medications) was used to reduce the blood pressure. Subsequently, minoxidil, 20 mg per day, was added to the regimen, and at this point, about 10 days after hospitalization, nitroprusside was discontinued. The blood pressure was approximately 170/100 mm Hg, i.e., the same level as on admission.

Discussion

This case exemplifies several points, including the inappropriate alteration of the medical regimen of a patient with a history of difficult-to-control hypertension. Of note, the patient probably had renovascular hypertension, which is a frequent cause of refractory hypertension. Nevertheless, although one might have hoped for better control, the baseline level of 170/100 mm Hg could not really have been considered poor control, especially in the absence of symptoms. This raises the question of whether any major adjustment of medications was advisable. Furthermore, before hospitalization, neither the clonidine nor the minoxidil doses were maximal, and increases in their dosages might have sufficed to reduce the blood pressure into the desired range. Alternatively, a beta-blocker might have been added to the regimen.

We have seen a hospitalized dialysis patient recently whose hypertension was resistant to 60 mg per day of minoxidil who became normotensive without side effects when the minoxidil dose was cautiously increased to a level as high as 125 mg per day for two days and then gradually reduced. Finally, in a patient with a prior history of hypertensive crises it was not wise to withdraw clonidine over a short interval at the same time that another major antihypertensive, minoxidil, was abruptly discontinued. One cannot predict in advance that captopril will be effective, even if the PRA is known to be elevated. In fact, there is some preliminary evidence that many patients whose hypertension is refractory to minoxidil will not respond to captopril. Whether the patient developed true rebound hypertension after withdrawal of medication or whether withdrawal simply unmasked the severity of his underlying untreated blood pressure cannot be said with certainty. Clonidine should have been reinstituted when the blood pressure rose strikingly.

If there had been evidence of a true hypertensive crisis, the alpha-adrenergic inhibitor phentolamine should also have been given intravenously.

In summary, inappropriate abrupt alteration of the medical regimen in a patient with reasonably well-controlled hypertension led to a hazardous deterioration of ccntrol and a prolonged, costly hospitalization.

CASE 18 CLONIDINE LOADING

A 45-year-old obese man with a long history of moderately severe hypertension without complications had taken no medications for several months because his physician wanted to evaluate the effect of weight loss and exercise. In a podiatry clinic, he asked if his blood pressure might be taken, and it was found to be 220/145 mm Hg, prompting immediate hospitalization. Physical examination revealed marked atherosclerotic changes in the fundal vessels and cardiomegaly without findings of congestive heart failure. Two hours after admission the blood pressure was approximately the same as that noted before admission, and it did not change with postural alteration. Laboratory data indicated grossly normal renal function.

The patient was given 40 mg of furosemide and 0.2 mg of clonidine. Clonidine was then given hourly at a dosage of 0.1 mg. The patient was kept supine. After the fourth hour the blood pressure had declined to 165/100 mm Hg. The regimen was then changed to chlorthalidone, 50 mg a day, and clonidine, 0.3 mg twice daily, and the patient was discharged 24 hours later with a stable blood pressure of 160/98 mm Hg. One week later hydralazine was added, 25 mg twice daily for two days, then 50 mg twice daily. Within five days the blood pressure was reduced to 140/85 mm Hg.

Discussion

Noncompliance and sometimes, as in this patient, withdrawal of therapy, account for a goodly number of episodes of severe hypertension. In a patient with a history of severe hypertension, one should not stop medications while awaiting the potential benefit of nonpharmacologic methods. In spite of the frighteningly high blood pressure recorded in this patient, he was not experiencing a true hypertensive crisis (there was no evidence of acute end-organ dysfunction) (see pp. 17–19). Therefore, parenteral therapy with nitroprusside or diazoxide was not indicated and might have produced untoward effects. Rather, the patient was managed with a newly recommended regimen that we have found to have a high rate of efficacy: sequential hourly administration of small doses of clonidine. Robinson et al. reported that 36 of 38 patients treated with this protocol had their diastolic blood pressure reduced to 110 mm Hg or less (from a mean of 139 mm Hg) within a six-hour period. None had important side effects. This method should be used only when the long-range plan includes the use of clonidine; otherwise withdrawal might lead to a return of severe hypertension. As would be expected, after the acute phase of therapy many patients require the addition of a diuretic and another antihypertensive medication (Step-3 agent). The combination of a long-acting diuretic (e.g., chlorthalidone), a sympatholytic agent (e.g., clonidine), and a vasodilator (e.g., hydralazine) has much to recommend it in a patient with severe hypertension.

CASE 19 TREATMENT OF HYPERTENSIVE CRISIS

An anuric 37-year-old patient receiving chronic hemodialysis, whose renal insufficiency probably resulted from long-standing severe essential hypertension, was admitted to the MICU at 11:00 PM with a blood pressure of 240/160 mm Hg, tachycardia, papilledema, distended neck veins, and frank pulmonary edema. He had gone to a wedding feast and missed his dialysis appointment the preceding day. His medications had included minoxidil, propranolol, and digoxin. The patient was treated with oxygen, morphine, and rotating tourniquets. Nitroprusside infusion was begun. The blood pressure decreased to 200/115 mm Hg, but there was only moderate improvement in the dyspnea, which remained severe. The nephrologist was called in and initiated ultrafiltration at 3:00 AM, with removal of two liters of fluid in 90 minutes. This resulted in marked improvement in symptoms and a further decline in blood pressure to 175/98 mm Hg. The patient was discharged from the hospital three days later with pressure of 160/90 mm Hg, using a regimen of clonidine and minoxidil.

Discussion

This patient experienced a true hypertensive crisis (pulmonary edema plus extreme hypertension). The precipitating factor probably was an expansion of the extracellular fluid by dietary indiscretion and missed dialysis. Of course, the extremely high blood pressure contributed to the pulmonary edema, and the latter would not be expected to respond to any therapy unless the blood pressure were reduced. Propranolol therapy, with its anti-inotropic effect, might have also predisposed the patient to congestive heart failure. Of interest, minoxidil has recently been shown, like hydralazine, to have a beneficial effect on CHF (by reducing afterload).

Nitroprusside, with its beneficial influence on both cardiac preload and afterload, was the parenteral drug of choice. Although diazoxide might also have improved the hemodynamic milieu by reducing the blood pressure, it would not have predictably ameliorated the CHF; and if it induced increased tachycardia, the cardiac status might have deteriorated.

The beneficial and well-tolerated influence of fluid removal by ultrafiltration (without dialysis) confirmed the role of volume expansion in the pathogenesis of both the pulmonary edema and the hypertensive crisis itself. Because of the episode of severe congestive heart failure, the medical regimen on discharge included clonidine instead of propranolol. This sympatholytic agent has been shown to adequately replace beta-blocker in patients receiving minoxidil.

CASE 20 DIABETES, HYPERTENSION, AND BETA-BLOCKERS

The antihypertensive regimen of a 43-year-old, insulin-requiring diabetic man with a childhood history of asthma (and no attacks since age 13) consisted of chlorthalidone, 50 mg once a day, and metoprolol, 50 mg twice daily. In order to obtain better blood pressure control, the dosage of the latter was doubled. Two weeks later the patient noted mild wheezing, which disappeared with the initiation of albuterol therapy. The physician noted that the patient's diabetic control (as manifested by increasing glucosuria and moderate increases in blood glucose) had deteriorated subsequent to initiation of antihypertensive therapy. He obtained some laboratory data, which were as follows: Na, 139 mEq/L; K, 3.3 mEq/L; Cl, 106 mEq/L; HCO_3, 21 mEq/L; BUN, 20 mg/dl; glucose 260 mg/dl (fasting). Because he was concerned that diuretic-induced hypokalemia may have contributed to the worsening of carbohydrate metabolism, the physician replaced the chlorthalidone with triamterene, 50 mg twice daily. Two weeks later, despite his wife's advice and urging, the patient participated in a matutinal 10-mile marathon jog sponsored by his church. For fear of developing hypoglycemia, he took no insulin before the race.

After four miles the patient noted marked generalized weakness, and he collapsed into the arms of an onlooker. On arrival at the nearest emergency room, he was noted to have slow respiration, flaccid muscles, and absent deep-tendon reflexes. The pulse rate was 45 beats per minute; blood pressure 140/85 mm Hg. Analysis of venous serum revealed the following: Na, 139 mEq/L; K, 9.3 mEq/L; Cl, 114 mEq/L; HCO_3, 13 mEq/L; BUN, 25 mg/dl; glucose 500 mg/dl; ketones, negative. An electrocardiogram showed atrial asystole, markedly peaked T-waves, and widening of the QRS complexes. The patient was treated with calcium chloride, $NaHCO_3$, and insulin intravenously, and was given sodium polystyrene sulfonate (Kayexalate) enemas. Over a period of several hours the ECG reverted to normal, and he recovered without complications.

Discussion

This complex case history is presented to emphasize the potential for uncommon but severe side effects when antihypertensive agents are used in an inappropriate setting. First, as indicated by the manufacturer of both cardioselective and noncardioselective beta-adrenergic inhibitors, it is best not to use these medications at all in patients with a history of bronchospastic disorders, even when there has been a long symptom-free interval. Of course, if beta blockers are to be ordered for such patients, it is best to use one of the cardioselective drugs, such as metoprolol or atenolol. Nevertheless, even these drugs carry the potential to induce or exacerbate bronchospasm in the predisposed individual, especially at higher dosage. In such patients they should be always be used together with a sympathomimetic bronchodilator medication. In the patient under discussion, bronchospasm occurred when the total daily dose of metoprolol was increased from 100 mg to 200 mg; the addition of the beta-stimulatory bronchodilator albuterol resulted in the disappearance of symptoms.

Beta-adrenergic inhibitors also have the potential to perturb carbohydrate homeostasis in patients with diabetes mellitus. Not only may they partially mask the admonitory symptoms of hypoglycemia (the tachycardia and palpitations, but not the sweating), but by inhibiting insulin release they may cause increasing hyperglycemia and, very rarely, produce hyperglycemic nonketotic coma. Of note, if hypoglycemia occurs in a patient receiving a beta-adrenergic inhibitor, the compensatory release of epinephrine by the adrenal medulla may result in a relatively unopposed alpha receptor–mediated vasoconstrictor response, with subsequent paradoxical hypertension, reflex bradycardia, and peripheral cyanosis. Although cardioselective agents have less propensity than nonselective agents such as propranolol, nadolol, or timolol to disturb carbohydrate homeostasis, the difference (as with their bronchial effects) appears to be relative and dose related.

Diuretic administration may on occasion also cause worsening of diabetic control. Frequently, this results from the adverse influence of potassium depletion, which can be reversed with potassium supplementation, but it may also relate to thiazide-induced inhibition of pancreatic insulin release. All of the sulfonamyl-containing diuretics (thiazides, chlorthalidone, metolazone, and furosemide) have the potential to influence diabetic control.

Perhaps the most important lesson to be learned from the case under discussion is that some patients with diabetes are at risk of developing severe hyperkalemia, particularly when multiple causative factors coexist (see Chapter 6). In the present case, these factors included the administration of a potassium-sparing diuretic (generally contraindicated in insulin-requiring diabetic patients), a beta-blocker (inhibition of the autonomic nervous system may impair internal potassium balance), insulin lack (which impairs internal potassium balance), exhaustive exercise (which causes a release of potassium from exercising muscle groups), and hyperosmolality (which impairs internal potassium balance).

In addition, many diabetic patients, especially those with renal insufficiency, albeit mild, have hyporeninemic hypoaldosteronism. In our patient, these problems resulted in a near-fatal hyperkalemic crisis.

CASE 21   SALT INTAKE AND THIAZIDE TREATMENT

A colleague of ours, a 46-year-old nephrologist, was begun by his physician on chlorthalidone, 50 mg once a day, for the treatment of essential hypertension. His untreated blood pressures were in the range of 150–170/95–100 mm Hg. After four weeks, the blood pressure averaged approximately 140/90 mm Hg but subsequently increased to about 160/95 mm Hg. After measuring his blood pressure one day, one of us queried the patient about his salt intake. He stated that he was being very careful about this, but when a 24-hour urine collection was obtained, the sodium excretion (and thus the dietary sodium intake) was noted to be 160 mEq, and the patient admitted to the habitual ingestion of a ham and cheese sandwich for lunch. Further dietary restriction resulted in improvement of blood pressure control.

Discussion

Since the antihypertensive action of diuretics is dependent upon their natriuretic properties, excessive sodium intake may obviate some or much of the beneficial effect of the medication. We present this case because it points out that even an authority in the area of renal sodium handling and edema may delude himself into the belief that his sodium intake has been appropriately curtailed. One hundred and sixty milliequivalents of sodium per day represents a value within the normal range of American dietary intake. It should be pointed out that the rather simple maneuver of collecting a 24-hour urine sample provides the clinician with an accurate assessment of salt ingestion and sometimes permits a beneficial alteration of the overall therapeutic regimen. Other considerations would have been an increase in the diuretic dosage or the addition of a Step-2 agent.

CASE 22   COMPLICATED HYPERTENSION: DECREASED RENAL FUNCTION

A 45-year-old man with a long-standing history of severe essential hypertension only poorly controlled despite several attempts at different drug regimens began to develop loss of renal function. The serum creatinine level was 2.3 mg/dl. Although his physician suspected that persistent blood pressure elevation was the proximate cause of the renal insufficiency, he was concerned that reduction of renal perfusion pressure might result in a further decline in GFR. Therefore, he made no changes in the patient's treatment program, which consisted of chlorthalidone, 50 mg once daily; propranolol, 160 mg twice daily; and prazosin, 15 mg twice daily. The blood pressure usually was in the range of 185/110 mm Hg. Over the next four months the renal function continued to decrease, and the serum creatinine concentration increased to 4.1 mg/dl. Trace pedal edema was observed. A nephrologist was consulted who recommended hospitalization and replacement of chlorthalidone with furosemide, 80 mg twice daily, and of the hydralazine with minoxidil, initially at a dose of 2.5 mg twice a day. Within five days, the use of a total daily dose of 5 mg of minoxidil caused the blood pressure to decrease to 135/85 mm Hg without symptoms or postural change. During the same interval, the serum creatinine increased from 4.1 to 5.8 mg/dl, and within another two weeks reached a level of 8.4 mg/dl. Dialysis was performed on two occasions. Afterward, over a period of approximately two months, the serum creatinine level gradually declined to the range of 2.8 mg/dl.

Discussion

The patient had what is often termed *complicated hypertension*—hypertension complicated by end-organ dysfunction, in this case decreased renal function probably related to arteriolonephrosclerosis (see Chapter 12). The crucial point to emphasize here is that the blood pressure in this type of patient must be controlled! If less than adequate control is accepted, the eventual outcome will be severe renal failure or some other catastrophe. Although normalization or near normalization of the pressure may (as happened in his case) result in exacerbation of renal failure, eventually renal function will stabilize and often improve. Even if hemodialysis is temporarily necessary, this is definitely preferable to complacency, with inadequate control of severe hypertension. Another point is that as renal function deteriorates (perhaps when the serum creatinine concentration exceeds 2.0 mg/dl and creatinine clearance decreases to less than 40 ml/min) a thiazide type of diuretic may not suffice, and a loop-type diuretic such as furosemide is frequently required. Of course, the marked sodium-retaining effect of minoxidil almost always mandates the use of furosemide at a substantial dosage.

CASE 23 RENOVASCULAR HYPERTENSION

A 48-year-old man with a history of easily controlled hypertension for more than nine years suddenly (over an eight-week period) developed accelerated and uncontrollable hypertension with blood pressures in the range of 240/140 mm Hg, and grade III retinopathy. The BUN was 18 mg/dl and the serum creatinine 1.1 mg/dl. A right-sided abdominal bruit with both systolic and diastolic components was noted. Arteriography revealed near-total stenosis of the right renal artery with poststenotic dilation. Renal venous renin was suppressed on the left side (the concentration was less than that in the inferior vena cava), and the ratio of right renal vein renin to left renal vein renin was 2.1. An aortorenal bypass graft was inserted. Four months after surgery, the blood pressure was 140/90 mm Hg. The serum creatinine was 1.0 mg/dl.

Discussion

This case illustrates a number of important features of renovascular hypertension. A sudden acceleration of previously controlled hypertension is one of the occurrences that should alert the clinician to the possibility that renovascular hypertension may have become superimposed upon essential hypertension. The presence of an abdominal bruit with systolic and diastolic components suggests strongly that turbulence secondary to stenosis of the renal artery is present. To assess the hemodynamic significance of the renal artery stenosis, renal venous PRA should be measured. The documentation of a ratio of affected side to unaffected side exceeding 1.5 is thought by many to indicate a physiologically significant renal artery stenosis. Suppression of renin secretion in the contralateral kidney has been proposed by several clinicians as one of the prognostic determinants of "cure."

CASE 24 RENOVASCULAR HYPERTENSION

A 58-year-old man with a history of long-standing hypertension was evaluated for renovascular hypertension. The patient was noted to have an elevated blood pressure while still in high school and had been treated with various regimens throughout the subsequent 40 years. He was readmitted for evaluation of his poorly controlled blood pressure. He volunteered a history of angina and intermittent claudication. The blood pressure was 230/120 mm Hg in both upper extremities. Fundoscopic examination revealed marked arteriolar narrowing. Bruits were present over both carotid arteries. The heart was significantly enlarged, with the point of maximum impulse deviated to the left. The serum creatinine concentration was 2.3 mg/dl.

The patient underwent a number of diagnostic studies, including an infusion pyelogram disclosing reduction in the size of the right kidney (10 cm) compared with a left kidney measuring 14.2 cm. The following day an aortogram with selective renal arteriograms was performed. These studies disclosed extensive atheromatous involvement of the aorta and an 80 per cent occlusion of the right renal artery. There was evidence of significant collateral flow to the lower pole of the right kidney. Renal vein renin levels were determined, disclosing a right renal vein plasma renin activity of 56 ng/ml/hr and a left renal vein PRA of 13.6 ng/ml/hr. The PRA from the inferior vena cava was 13.7 ng/ml/hr.

Discussion

This case raises a number of questions that should be considered:

1. Is the hypertension in this patient of a renovascular etiology?
2. If it is of a renovascular etiology, is it of a curable form?
3. If the above questions are answered in the affirmative, should we proceed with surgery?

The ratio of the right and left renal vein PRA values markedly exceeds 1:5, which indicates that ischemia of the right kidney has contributed to the patient's hypertension.

The abnormal serum creatinine concentration and the fact that the PRA of the effluent from the left renal vein renin was not suppressed below that of the IVP suggests that there are irreversible secondary changes in the "normal" contralateral (left) kidney that would militate against a "cure" should nephrectomy be carried out on the right. Laragh has proposed that in curable hypertension, one should anticipate not only a elevated renin level on the affected side, but a suppressed renin level on the contralateral side.

Finally, significant target organ involvement, which has already been sustained by the patient (hypertensive cardiovascular disease manifested by left ventricular hypertrophy), and our knowledge that he has extensive atheromatous involvement of major segments of the arterial tree, as manifested by the carotid bruits and the history of intermittent claudication, suggest that he is an extremely poor surgical risk.

The major point in this case is that since the patient presented with evidence of extensive atheromatous disease, which militated against surgical intervention, an extensive, expensive (and occasionally morbid) diagnostic evaluation should not have been undertaken. Rather, the patient's medical management should have been pressed more rigorously. An additional consideration is the possible role of transluminal angioplasty in such a patient.

CASE 25 HYPERTENSION WITH HYPOKALEMIC METABOLIC ALKALOSIS

A 46-year-old man complained of severe weakness of the extremities of two weeks' duration, which had markedly worsened during the last two days. He stated that he used no medications or remedies and that his health had always been excellent.

Physical examination showed an anxious man with profound muscular weakness. His blood pressure was 148/95 mm Hg, and his pulse 110 beats per minute with an occasional premature contraction. The muscles of the leg and thigh were slightly tender; ankle and knee jerks were present, but diminished. The sensory examination was normal.

Pertinent laboratory findings included a serum potassium of 1.2 mEq/L; sodium, 147 mEq/L; chloride, 100 mEq/L; and bicarbonate, 37 mEq/L. The serum creatine phosphokinase activity was markedly elevated (21,000 IU/L). The urine showed a specific gravity of 1.007 and a moderately positive dipstick reaction for heme pigment. His ECG revealed a normal sinus rhythm with occasional multifocal premature ventricular contractions and very prominent U waves.

Additionally, it was noted that the PRA was undetectable and the plasma aldosterone concentration abnormally low. Before potassium administration, a spot urine sample showed a potassium concentration of 45 mEq/L and a chloride level of 30 mEq/L.

Discussion

This patient's condition illustrates the association of hypertension with hypokalemic metabolic alkalosis. The findings of moderate hypertension, hypernatremia, hypokalemic metabolic alkalosis with a urinary chloride concentration greater than 20 mEq/L, and renal potassium wasting suggested the presence of mineralocorticoid excess. If the patient had primary aldosteronism, his plasma aldosterone value should have been distinctly elevated, usually coupled with a very low value for PRA. Because both aldosterone and PRA were suppressed, it was likely that the patient was either ingesting or producing a substance other than aldosterone with mineralocorticoid activity. Repeat questioning disclosed that he habitually ingested large amounts of candy containing licorice.

Licorice contains glycyrrhizinic acid, which acts on the renal tubule in a manner identical to that of aldosterone. Many cases of hypertension with hypokalemic metabolic alkalosis and low values for renin and aldosterone have been observed in patients who consume large amounts of licorice. Although candy has been the main source (it should be noted that now many "licorice-type" candies actually do not contain licorice), chewing tobacco has also been reported to constitute a source of licorice sufficient to produce a syndrome simulating primary aldosteronism.

CASE 26   HYPERTENSION WITH HYPOKALEMIA

A 71-year-old retired laborer with established moderate hypertension of long duration sought medical advice because of the recent onset of weakness of the lower extremities. The patient's hypertension was well controlled for the past four years with a thiazide-type diuretic and hydralazine.

Laboratory evaluation revealed marked hypokalemia (2.2 mEq/L). A review of the patient's medical records disclosed that routine serial laboratory determinations over the past three years (obtained during the administration of the antihypertensive regimen described above), consistently disclosed serum potassium levels that were in the low normal range.

Discussion

Initially, it was unclear how the patient remained on the same regimen for many years without developing hypokalemia until his current illness. This issue was clarified by a careful dietary history. It revealed that during the preceding year the patient's dental problems became progressively more serious, eventually resulting in an edentulous state. As a result, his dietary intake had been largely limited to soft, processed foods, particularly bread pudding. The dietitian estimated that his daily potassium intake seldom, if ever, exceeded 20 mEq/day, which is at least three to five times lower than the normal level. It was assumed that the recent inadequate potassium intake fell short of the amount the patient was excreting under the influence of the medication-induced increase in aldosterone levels, and that a cumulative negative potassium balance ensued.

Appendix 1

SODIUM AND POTASSIUM CONTENT OF COMMON FOODS

The two parts of this appendix, A and B, provide information on the sodium and potassium content of various food items. This information is drawn from the following sources:

1. Pennington, JAT, and Church, HN: Food Values of Portions Commonly Used, 13th ed. Harper & Row, New York, 1980.
2. Adams, CF: Nutritive Value of American Foods. Agriculture Handbook No. 456. Agricultural Research Service, U.S. Department of Agriculture, Washington, D.C., 1975.

Some products vary considerably in their sodium content. This appendix provides some representative values. These reflect current processing practices and typical product formulas. Should these methods of preparation change, sodium values may change also.

A. REPRESENTATIVE DIETARY SOURCES WITH A LOW SODIUM AND HIGH POTASSIUM CONTENT (AVERAGE VALUES)

Food Item	Amount	Potassium		Sodium	
		mg	mEq	mg	mEq
FRUIT AND FRUIT JUICES					
Apples					
Fresh	1 med.	165	4	1	<0.1
Juice	4 oz.	125	3	1.3	<0.1
Apricots					
Fresh	2–3	281	7	1	<0.1
Canned	3 halves	234	6	1	<0.1
Avocados (3¼" × 4")	½	604	15	4	0.2
Bananas (6" long), small	1	370	9	1	<0.1
Cherries, fresh	½ cup	191	5	2	0.1
Currants	¾ cup	257	7	2	0.1
Grapefruit					
Fresh	½ med.	135	3	1	<0.1
Juice	4 oz.	200	5	1	<0.1
Guavas	1 med.	289	7	4	0.2
Mangoes	½ med.	189	5	7	0.3
Melons (5" diam.)					
Cantaloupe	¼	251	6	12	0.5
Honeydew	¼	251	6	12	0.5
Oranges					
Fresh	1 small	200	5	1	<0.1
Juice	4 oz.	250	7	1.5	<0.1
Peaches, fresh	1 med.	202	5	1	<0.1
Pears					
Fresh	½ med.	130	3	2	0.1
Canned	2 halves	84	2	1	<0.1
Pineapples					
Fresh	½ cup	113	3	1	<0.1
Canned	½ cup	122	3	1	<0.1
Juice	4 oz.	186	5	1	<0.1
Plums, fresh	2 med.	299	8	2	0.1

A. REPRESENTATIVE DIETARY SOURCES WITH A LOW SODIUM AND HIGH POTASSIUM CONTENT (AVERAGE VALUES) *(Continued)*

Food Item	Amount	Potassium mg	mEq	Sodium mg	mEq
Prunes					
Dried or cooked	4 med.	329	8	4	0.2
Juice	4 oz.	282	7	3	0.1
Raspberries	1 cup	255	6	1	<0.1
Strawberries	1 cup	268	7	1	<0.1
VEGETABLES (Cooked Without Salt)					
Asparagus, fresh or frozen	6 spears	239	6	2	0.1
Beans, dry					
White, cooked	½ cup	416	11	7	0.3
Red, kidney	⅖ cup	340	9	3	0.1
Lima, cooked	⅝ cup	422	11	1	<0.1
Broccoli, fresh or frozen	1 large stalk	267	7	10	0.4
Brussels sprouts	6–7 sprouts	273	7	10	0.4
Cauliflower	⅞ cup	207	5	10	0.4
Corn, cooked (4″ long)	1 ear	196	5	Trace	Trace
Lettuce, iceberg	3½ oz.	264	7	9	0.4
Peas, fresh or frozen	⅔ cup	196	5	1	<0.1
Peppers, green, raw	1 med.	129	3	Trace	Trace
Potatoes					
Boiled	1 small	285	7	2	0.1
Sweet, canned	1 small	120	3	48	2
Tomatoes					
Raw	1 med.	366	9	4	0.2
Juice, low sodium	4 oz.	276	7	4	0.2
CEREAL AND STARCHES (Cooked Without Salt)					
Macaroni, noodles, spaghetti	1 cup	82	2	2	0.1
Oatmeal, cooked	1 cup	130	3	1	<0.1
Wheat germ	3 tbsp.	232	6	1	<0.1
MEAT, FISH, POULTRY (Cooked Without Salt)					
Beef					
Hamburger	4 oz.	382	10	41	2
Chuck, cooked	3 oz.	310	8	44	2
Liver, cooked	3½ oz.	325	8	86	4
Round, cooked	3 oz.	344	9	58	3
Sirloin	4 oz.	273	7	29	1
Chicken, cooked	3½ oz.	320	8	78	3
Lamb, leg, roast	3½ oz.	246	6	41	2
Pork					
Loin and chops	3 oz.	233	6	51	2
Ham, fresh	3 oz.	220	6	43	2
Tuna, canned in water, low sodium	3½ oz.	279	7	41	2
Veal, cutlet	3 oz.	258	7	56	2
MISCELLANEOUS					
Coffee, black	8 oz.	90	2	—	Trace
Tea	8 oz.	113	3	—	Trace
Salt substitute	½ tsp.	1368	35	—	Trace

B. HIGH-SODIUM DIETARY SOURCES (AVERAGE VALUES)

Food Item*	Amount	Sodium mg	Sodium mEq	Potassium mg	Potassium mEq
VEGETABLES					
Sauerkraut, canned	⅔ cup	747	32	140	4
Tomato juice, canned	6 oz.	360	16	408	10
Tomato puree, canned	4 oz.	1000	43	1060	27
Tomato sauce, canned	4 oz.	656	29	463	12
Vegetables, packaged in a sauce (e.g., green beans in a mushroom sauce)	3½ oz.	364	16	150	4
Vegetables, canned (e.g., carrots, drained)	3½ oz.	236	10	120	3
GRAIN PRODUCTS					
Cereals, instant, cooked (e.g., Quaker oatmeal)	½ cup	215	9	92	2
Crackers and snack foods					
Butter thins	1	306	13	32	1
Cheese Tid-Bits, Nabisco	10	164	7	9	0.2
Corn chips, Fritos	1 oz.	202	9	23	0.6
Pretzels	1	218	9	17	0.4
Popcorn, salted	1 cup	116	5	28	0.7
Potato chips	1 oz., or 10	252	1	196	5
Saltines	2	66	3	7	0.3
Saltines, with unsalted tops	2	50	1	196	5
MEATS AND FISH					
Anchovies		N/A†	N/A	N/A	N/A
Bacon, cured, broiled	1 strip, 1 oz.	76	3	17	0.4
Beef, dried, chipped	3 oz.	3660	159	170	4
Bologna	1 oz.	364	16	64	2
Canned meats (e.g., boned chicken)	3½ oz.	543	24	138	3
Caviar, sturgeon, granular	1 tsp.	220	10	18	0.5
Cheeses (e.g., processed American)	1 oz.	318	14	22	0.6
Corned beef, cooked	3½ oz.	1740	76	150	6
Crab, canned or cooked	3 oz.	850	37	94	4
Fish, frozen breaded (e.g., shrimp)	3½ oz.	537	23	99	4
Frankfurter, cooked	1	542	24	108	5
Ham, cured butt, cooked	3½ oz.	718	31	332	8
Herring, salted or smoked		N/A	N/A	N/A	N/A
Kosher meats		N/A	N/A	N/A	N/A
Luncheon meats (e.g., Oscar Meyer ham and cheese loaf)	1 slice	372	16	80	3
Salt pork, raw	1 oz.	339	15	12	0.3
Sardines, in oil	3½ oz.	510	22	560	14
Sausage (e.g., pork links)	3½ oz.	740	32	140	4
Shellfish (e.g., oysters, fried)	3 oz.	206	9	203	0.2
Smoked fish		N/A	N/A	N/A	N/A
Smoked meats		N/A	N/A	N/A	N/A
BEVERAGES					
Buttermilk (whole milk)	1 cup	212	9	388	10
Cocoa mix, instant, Nestles	1 oz.	141	6	347	9

*Because similar food items produced by different manufacturers vary in their sodium content, we have, where appropriate, included the sodium content of a representative brand.

†N/A, not available.

B. HIGH-SODIUM DIETARY SOURCES (AVERAGE VALUES) *(Continued)*

Food Item*	Amount	Sodium mg	Sodium mEq	Potassium mg	Potassium mEq
SEASONINGS					
Monosodium glutamate, Accent	1 tbsp.	62	7	N/A	N/A
Barbecue sauce, Open Pit	1 tbsp.	213	9	6	0.1
Bouillon (e.g., beef)	1 cube	960	41	4	0.1
Broth, instant, dry (e.g., beef)	1 tbsp.	3611	157	N/A	N/A
Catsup	1 tbsp.	156	7	55	1
Celery salt		N/A	N/A	N/A	N/A
Chili sauce	1 tbsp.	228	10	63	2
Garlic salt		N/A	N/A	N/A	N/A
Gravy, brown, Knorr-Swiss	1 tbsp.	441	19	70	2
Meat tenderizer, Adolph's	1 tbsp.	1745	76	Trace	Trace
Mustard, yellow	1 tsp.	63	3	7	0.2
Onion salt		N/A	N/A	N/A	N/A
Salt (NaCl)	1 tsp.	1955	85	Trace	Trace
Sea salt		N/A	N/A	N/A	N/A
Steak sauce, Lea & Perrins	1 tbsp.	149	6	64	2
Soy sauce	1 tbsp.	858	37	54	1
Tartar sauce	1 tbsp.	141	6	16	0.4
Worcestershire sauce	1 tsp.	49	2	40	1
MISCELLANEOUS					
Baking powder, home use, straight phosphate	1 tsp.	247	11	5	0.1
Baking soda	1 tsp.	821	36	N/A	N/A
Combination foods					
Frozen dinners (e.g., fried chicken, Swanson)	1 meal	1173	51	731	19
Frozen pizza (e.g., sausage, Celeste)	1 slice	581	25	246	6
Pot pies (e.g., turkey)	1 pie	864	38	259	7
Dips (e.g., French onion, Sealtest)	1 tsp.	84	4	26	0.7
Flour, self-rising, wheat	⅞ cup, sifted	1079	47	90	2
Gatorade, citrus	1 cup	123	5	23	0.6
Nuts, salted (e.g., peanuts)	3½ oz.	460	20	700	18
Olives, green, pickled	2 med.	312	14	7	0.2
Pickles, dill	1 large	1428	62	200	5
Pickle relish, sweet	1 tbsp.	107	5	N/A	N/A
Seaweed, kelp, raw	3½ oz.	3007	131	5273	135
Soups (e.g., chicken noodle)	1 serv., 7 oz.	754	33	40	1
Salad dressing, Italian	1 tbsp.	293	13	2	<0.1

*Because similar food items produced by different manufacturers vary in their sodium content, we have, where appropriate, included the sodium content of a representative brand.

†N/A, not available.

Appendix 2

ACCEPTABLE LOW-SODIUM FLAVORING AIDS

Spices: Allspice, cardamom, cinnamon, cloves, curry, ginger, mace, mustard, nutmeg, paprika, various peppers, saffron, turmeric

Herbs: Basil, bay leaf, chives, fennel, marjoram, mint, oregano, rosemary, sage, savory, tarragon, thyme

Extracts: Almond, lemon, maple, orange, peppermint, rum, strawberry, raspberry, vanilla

Seeds: Anise, caraway, dill, poppy seed, sesame

Other: Cocoa (not Dutch process), garlic, green pepper, fresh horseradish, leeks, lemon juice, onion, orange peel, parsley, sugar (a small amount of sugar added to vegetables during cooking helps to bring out natural flavors)

Modified from Salmon, MB, and Quigley, AE: Enjoying Your Restricted Diet. Charles C Thomas, Springfield, Ill., 1972.

Appendix 3

FIXED-DOSE COMBINATION ANTIHYPERTENSIVE DRUGS

A. DIURETIC-DIURETIC COMBINATIONS

Product and Distributor	Diuretic	Diuretic	CI*
Moduretic (MSD)	5 mg amiloride	50 mg hydrochloro-thiazide	20
Spironolactone w/ Hydrochlorothiazide (Various)	25 mg spironolac-tone	25 mg hydrochloro-thiazide	6+
Spironolactone w/ Hydrochlorothiazide (Rugby)	As above	As above	8
Spironolactone w/ Hydrochlorothiazide (Geneva Generics)	As above	As above	12
Spironolactone w/ Hydrochlorothiazide (Lederle)	As above	As above	18
Aldactazide (Searle)	As above	As above	20
Spiractazide (Three P)	As above	As above	12
Spironazide (Schein)	As above	As above	7
Dyazide (SKF)	50 mg triamterene	As above	11

*The *cost index* (CI), based on the cost per capsule or tablet and located on the right side of the product listings, is a ratio of the average wholesale price for equivalent quantities of a drug. It is designed to help quickly determine the relative costs of similar or identical products, but is not a dollar and cents figure. For example, if the cost index figures of a group of products range from 3 to 18, the most expensive product costs six times more than the least expensive product.

A cost index of 3+ for generic products (various) indicates that the least expensive generic product has a cost index of 3; however, the "+" means that other generic products may be more expensive. This does not mean that all generic products are less expensive than the brand name products.

The cost indices for dosage forms of different strengths are adjusted to permit comparison of equivalent amounts of products.

All tables in Appendix 3 modified with permission from Facts and Comparisons, May 1983.

B. DIURETICS PLUS RAUWOLFIA DERIVATIVES

Product and Distributor	Diuretic	Rauwolfia Derivative	CI*
Chlorothiazide w/Reserpine Tablets (Various)	500 mg chlorothiazide	0.125 mg reserpine	120+
Diupres 500 Tablets (MSD)	As above	As above	200
Chlorothiazide w/Reserpine Tablets (Various)	250 mg chlorothiazide	As above	44+
Chloroserpine-250 Tablets (Various)	As above	As above	46+
Diupres 250 Tablets (MSD)	As above	As above	128
Serpasil-Esidrix #2 Tablets (Ciba)	50 mg hydrochlorothiazide	0.1 mg reserpine	195
Hydrochlorothiazide w/Reserpine Tablets (Various)	50 mg hydrochlorothiazide	0.125 mg reserpine	17+
Hydro Plus Tablets (Reid-Provident)	As above	As above	71
Hydropres 50 Tablets (MSD)	As above	As above	200
Hydro-Reserp Tablets (Camall)	As above	As above	41
Hydro-Serp Tablets (Various)	As above	As above	22+
Hydroserpine Tablets (Various)	As above	As above	22+
Hydrotensin-50 Tablets (Mayrand)	As above	As above	108
Serpasil-Esidrix #1 Tablets (Ciba)	25 mg hydrochlorothiazide	0.1 mg reserpine	127
Hydrochlorothiazide w/Reserpine Tablets (Various)	25 mg hydrochlorothiazide	0.125 mg reserpine	16+
Hydropres 25 Tablets (MSD)	As above	As above	128
Hydro-Serp Tablets (Various)	As above	As above	29+
Hydroserpine Tablets (Various)	As above	As above	20+
Mallopress Tablets (Mallard)	As above	As above	32
Diurese-R Tablets (American Urologicals)	4 mg trichlormethiazide	0.1 mg reserpine	187
Metatensin #4 Tablets (Merrell Dow)	As above	As above	381
Naquival Tablets (Schering)	As above	As above	306
Metatensin #2 Tablets (Merrell Dow)	2 mg trichlormethiazide	As above	255
Diutensen-R Tablets (Wallace)	2.5 mg methyclothiazide	As above	485
Hydromox R Tablets (Lederle)	50 mg quinethazone	0.125 mg reserpine	538
Salutensin Tablets (Bristol Labs)	50 mg hydroflumethiazide	As above	379
Salutensin-Demi Tablets (Bristol Labs)	25 mg hydroflumethiazide	As above	295
Regroton Tablets (USV)	50 mg chlorthalidone	0.25 mg reserpine	377

B. DIURETICS PLUS RAUWOLFIA DERIVATIVES (Continued)

Product and Distributor	Diuretic	Rauwolfia Derivative	CI*
Demi-Regroton Tablets (USV)	25 mg chlorthalidone	0.125 mg reserpine	336
Renese-R Tablets (Pfizer)	2 mg polythiazide	0.25 mg reserpine	355
Rauzide Tablets (Squibb)	4 mg bendroflumethiazide	50 mg powdered rauwolfia serpentina	449
Enduronyl Tablets (Abbott)	5 mg methyclothiazide	0.25 mg deserpidine	344
Enduronyl Forte Tablets (Abbott)	5 mg methyclothiazide	0.5 mg deserpidine	393
Oreticyl 50 Tablets (Abbott)	50 mg hydrochlorothiazide	0.125 mg deserpidine	182
Oreticyl 25 Tablets (Abbott)	25 mg hydrochlorothiazide	As above	117
Oreticyl Forte Tablets (Abbott)	25 mg hydrochlorothiazide	0.25 mg deserpidine	164

*See footnote for Table A, p. 184.

C. DIURETICS–RAUWOLFIA DERIVATIVES PLUS ADDITIONAL AGENTS

Product and Distributor	Diuretic	Rauwolfia Derivative	Other Agent	CI*
Rautrax Tablets (Squibb)	400 mg flumethiazide	50 mg powdered rauwolfia serpentina	400 mg potassium chloride	581
Rautrax-N Tablets (Squibb)	4 mg bendroflumethiazide	50 mg powdered rauwolfia serpentina	As above	581
Cam-ap-es Tablets (Camall)	15 mg hydrochlorothiazide	0.1 mg reserpine	25 mg hydralazine HCl	63
Hydrap-Es Tablets (Lemmon)	As above	As above	As above	28
Hyserp Tablets (Reid-Provident)	As above	As above	As above	128
R-HCTZ-H Tablets (Lederle)	As above	As above	As above	156
Ser-A-Gen Tablets (Generix)	As above	As above	As above	57
Seralazide Tablets (Lannett)	As above	As above	As above	57
Ser-Ap-Es Tablets (Ciba)	As above	As above	As above	270
Ser-Hydra-Zine Tablets (Three P)	As above	As above	As above	28
Tri-Hydroserpine Tablets (Rugby)	As above	As above	As above	75
Unipres Tablets (Reid-Provident)	As above	As above	As above	216
Naturetin c̄ K 5 mg Tablets (Squibb)	5 mg bendroflumethiazide	As above	500 mg potassium chloride	385

*See footnote for Table A, p. 184.

D. DIURETICS PLUS ADDITIONAL AGENTS

Product and Distributor	Diuretic	Other Agent	CI*
Apresazide 100/50 Capsules (Ciba)	50 mg hydrochlorothiazide	100 mg hydralazine HCl	384
Apresazide 50/50 Capsules (Ciba)	50 mg hydrochlorothiazide	50 mg hydralazine HCl	315
Hydral 50/50 Capsules (Reid-Provident)	As above	As above	200
Apresazide 25/25 Capsules (Ciba)	As above	25 mg hydralazine HCl	211
Hydral 25/25 Capsules (Reid-Provident)	As above	As above	133
Apresodex Tablets (Rugby)	15 mg hydrochlorothiazide	As above	45
Apresoline-Esidrix Tablets (Ciba)	As above	As above	185
Inderide-80/25 Tablets (Ayerst)	25 mg hydrochlorothiazide	80 mg propranolol HCl	328
Inderide-40/25 Tablets (Ayerst)	25 mg hydrochlorothiazide	40 mg propranolol HCl	235
Timolide Tablets (MSD)	25 mg hydrochlorothiazide	10 mg timolol maleate	352
Aldoril D50 Tablets (MSD)	50 mg hydrochlorothiazide	500 mg methyldopa	453
Aldoril D30 Tablets (MSD)	30 mg hydrochlorothiazide	As above	422
Aldoril-25 Tablets (MSD)	25 mg hydrochlorothiazide	250 mg methyldopa	265
Aldoril-15 Tablets (MSD)	15 mg hydrochlorothiazide	As above	234
Aldoclor-250 Tablets (MSD)	250 mg chlorothiazide	As above	265
Aldoclor-150 Tablets (MSD)	150 mg chlorothiazide	As above	234
Esimil Tablets (Ciba)	25 mg hydrochlorothiazide	10 mg guanethidine monosulfate	378
Eutron Filmtabs (Abbott)	5 mg methyclothiazide	25 mg pargyline HCl	346
Diutensen Tablets (Wallace)	2.5 mg methyclothiazide	2 mg cryptenamine (as tannate)	415
Combipres 0.2 Tablets (Boehringer Ingelheim)	15 mg chlorthalidone	0.2 mg clonidine HCl	403
Combipres 0.1 Tablets (Boehringer Ingelheim)	15 mg chlorthalidone	0.1 mg clonidine HCl	315
Minizide 5 Capsules (Pfizer)	0.5 mg polythiazide	5 mg prazosin HCl	532
Minizide 2 Capsules (Pfizer)	0.5 mg polythiazide	2 mg prazosin HCl	351
Minizide 1 Capsules (Pfizer)	0.5 mg polythiazide	1 mg prazosin HCl	279

*See footnote for Table A, p. 184.

E. RAUWOLFIA DERIVATIVES PLUS ADDITIONAL AGENTS

Product and Distributor	Rauwolfia Derivative	Other Agent	CI*
Serpasil-Apresoline #2 Tablets (Ciba)	0.2 mg reserpine	50 mg hydralazine HCl	251
Dralserp Tablets (Lemmon)	0.1 mg reserpine	25 mg hydralazine HCl	75
Serpasil-Apresoline #1 Tablets As above (Ciba)	As above		182
Ruhexatal w/Reserpine Tablets (Lemmon)	As above	30 mg mannitol hexa-nitrate	73

*See footnote for Table A, p. 184.

Index

In this index, numbers in *italics* refer to illustrations; numbers followed by (t) refer to tables.